Praise for *Restore*

"*Restore: The Life-Changing Power of Right-Away Wellness*, by Jim Donnelly and Steve Welch, is a quick and practical guide on how to improve one's health. Presented by two successful entrepreneurs who have built the largest retail health company in the country, this book provides an amazing roadmap for what to do today to have a better life tomorrow. The authors took the complexities of our health and wellness and boiled them down into an understandable journey."

—Jake Arrieta, former Major League Baseball pitcher, World Series champion, and Cy Young Award winner

"*Restore: The Life-Changing Power of Right-Away Wellness* is a practical guide to achieving a state of hyper wellness. Jim Donnelly and Steve Welch's approach is both insightful and practical, providing actionable steps to unlock the body's full potential for health and vitality. Jim and Steve emphasize the importance of minimizing external interventions, while allowing the body to function as it was naturally designed to. The book is filled with evidence-based information on nutrition, exercise, and mindfulness, all aimed at helping individuals take charge of their well-being. Whether you're just starting your wellness journey or looking to take it to the next level, *Restore* is a powerful resource that will lead you to a healthier, more empowered life. I recommend *Restore* for anyone seeking to design a roadmap to optimal health."

—Tom Hale, CEO of Oura Ring

"*Restore: The Life-Changing Power of Right-Away Wellness*, by Jim Donnelly and Steve Welch, presents a groundbreaking approach to health and well-being, encompassing a diverse range of individuals, from professional athletes to everyday people facing various health challenges. The authors explore the potential benefits of immediate interventions, offering insights into how they can contribute to overall wellness and alleviate suffering. Backed by expert insights and inspiring stories, this book invites readers to consider the potential impact of immediate wellness strategies on their lives. Discover a journey toward better health and well-being through these pages."

—John Day, MD, author of *The AFib Cure* and *The Longevity Plan*

restore

THE
LIFE-CHANGING
POWER
OF RIGHT-AWAY
WELLNESS

Jim Donnelly
and Steve Welch

with Matthew D. LaPlante

BenBella Books, Inc.
Dallas, TX

BenBella Books, Inc.
10440 N. Central Expressway
Suite 800
Dallas, TX 75231
benbellabooks.com*
Send feedback to feedback@benbellabooks.com

BenBella is a federally registered trademark.

Printed in the United States of America
10 9 8 7 6 5 4 3 2 1

Library of Congress Control Number: 2023049240
ISBN 9781637745090 (hardcover)
ISBN 9781637745106 (electronic)

Editing by Claire Schulz
Copyediting by Karen Wise
Proofreading by Ashley Casteel and Rebecca Maines
Indexing by WordCo. Indexing Services
Text design and composition by Jordan Koluch
Cover design by Brigid Pearson
Logo and cover artwork courtesy of Restore Hyper Wellness
Printed by Lake Book Manufacturing

This book is dedicated to:

*The studio owners who have invested in
making positive impacts in their communities.*

*The Restore employees who work tirelessly to
expand the limits of personal health and performance.*

*The people from every walk of life who have
trusted us with their wellness journey.*

Contents

Authors' Note   ix

Introduction   xi

Index of Hyper Wellness Success   xxi

Chapter 1: Hyper Wellness   1

Chapter 2: Headwinds and Tailwinds   25

Chapter 3: Cold   53

Chapter 4: Heat   79

Chapter 5: Oxygen   97

Chapter 6: Hydration   119

Chapter 7: Rest   135

Chapter 8: Light   153

Chapter 9: Nourishment   177

Chapter 10: Movement   195

Chapter 11: Connection   215

Chapter 12: Watchpoints and Waypoints   227

Conclusion   245

Notes   249

Index   273

Authors' Note

The stories in this book are based on scores of interviews conducted with Restore clients who come from communities across the nation. In cases in which a person might reasonably be identifiable based on their story, we've chosen to change some pieces of biographical information—in many cases, simply their name and city—to protect their privacy. In no case, however, have we altered health results to make it seem as though someone had a more positive outcome than what actually happened to them, and others like them, in similar circumstances. Indeed, we've chosen to be very conservative about the client experiences we have included in this book and have declined to include any client whose story—however positive and compelling—is not well aligned to peer-reviewed studies that inform us of the sorts of outcomes that are actually likely.

Introduction

There was an older man in a brown checkered fedora and a younger woman with her teenaged son by her side. There was a middle-aged police officer who was just getting done with her overnight shift, and a twenty-something computer programmer getting ready to start his workday. There were two nurses, colleagues for decades, who were spending some time away from the hospital where they'd been on-shift or on-call for ten days straight.

It was a Tuesday morning in Austin, a few minutes before 10 a.m., and as we opened the door of the Restore Hyper Wellness studio on Aldrich Street, the regular crowd shuffled in.

This wasn't exactly what we thought our client base would look like when we opened our first studio, about nine miles southwest of this spot, back in 2015. At that time we figured the whole-body cryotherapy and other therapies we were providing would mostly be sought after by athletes, especially those who were starting to experience the slowing cycle of recovery that comes with aging.

That's how we'd fallen into this line of work. Neither of us were high-level athletes at that point in our lives, but we both liked to push ourselves. We'd been training together for a triathlon, and we were both pretty beaten up. Sore all day. Achy all over. Recovery taking longer and longer. A lot of people told us that's just the way it goes as you get older. We figured that was true.

But we would have done just about anything to feel better—even if it meant stripping down to our skivvies and getting blasted with jets of super-cold air, a practice growing trendier by the day in Austin in the mid-2010s. Whole-body cryotherapy was all the rage.

The "whole body" part of this sounded like a crazy fad, but cold therapy wasn't really a new idea. We both grew up in homes where "just put some ice on it" was the solution to most of life's bumps and bruises. And that's what a lot of people have been told for a very long time. One of the world's oldest known surgical texts, a 5,500-year-old Egyptian papyrus scroll known as the *Secret Book of the Physician*, made numerous references to using cold as a therapy. In one section, the hieroglyphics instruct a healer to tell a patient with a swollen, pus-filled lump in their chest, "I will treat [you] with cold applications to that abscess."[1]

A few thousand years later, in Greece, Hippocrates used cold therapy to treat his patients, too. These practices have continued in places around the world, mostly using ice and cold-water immersion. It wasn't until the middle of the last century, though, that we ingenious humans figured out a way to get ourselves even colder using air cooled with liquid nitrogen. In 1981, a health researcher named Toshiro Yamauchi, who had constructed a makeshift whole-body cryotherapy chamber at Reiken Rheumatism Village Institute in Oita, Japan, published the first scientific article on exposing his patients to short bursts of temperatures as low as negative 240 degrees Fahrenheit, which appeared to be an effective treatment for arthritis. Over the decades since, clinical studies have demonstrated whole-body cryo can be an effective treatment for alleviating asthma, slowing Alzheimer's disease, mitigating anxiety, decreasing chronic pain, minimizing migraines, and reducing the symptoms of multiple sclerosis, and the practice has picked up adherents around the world for many other conditions as well—especially those who use it for athletic recovery.[2]

Yet we'd never heard of it—not until Jim and his wife ran into a friend who was on her way to a lunchtime cryo session and invited them along.

"It's the craziest thing," she said. "You walk out feeling like a million bucks. You feel so energized."

Jim has always been an "I'll try anything once" kind of guy—a trait he'd honed over a career including Army service, entrepreneurship, and Fortune 100 corporate leadership—so he and his wife followed their friend to the spa, giggled as they took turns getting into a funny-looking metal tube, and shivered through the coldest three minutes of their lives.

> ### *"You walk out feeling like a million bucks.*
> ### *You feel so energized."*

Jim wasn't surprised he indeed felt a surge of energy when it was all over. That part of the experience made sense at a fundamental, biological level. Every thrill seeker is familiar with the rush that comes when an acutely stressful situation prompts their nervous system to secrete endorphins, which attach to the brain's opiate receptors, activating the release of dopamine, the so-called happiness hormone. In most cases that feeling comes along quickly and usually goes away after a few hours. But that night Jim realized he wasn't just feeling an endorphin rush. He also wasn't feeling the sort of pain he'd been experiencing—indeed that he'd gotten used to—since we'd started training together. The soreness in his muscles was gone. The aching in his joints was, too. And those feelings were still gone when we got together the next morning.

"It really *is* the craziest thing," he said. "You've got to try this."

On Hope and Hogwash

It took a few weeks before Steve was ready to give it a go. It wasn't that Jim's sudden enthusiasm wasn't compelling, but Steve's hard-won bullshit meter was spinning good and fast. As the founder of a firm that had funded hundreds of health-related start-ups, Steve was reviewing scores of venture funding proposals each week, and the ones that offer a lot in return for very little up front are usually hogwash. It seemed implausible that something done in just a few minutes could have such a profound impact for days and weeks to come. And if it worked as well as people were saying it did, wouldn't it already be in every doctor's office and hospital around the globe? Jim's excitement proved convincing, though. So did the peer-reviewed studies that Steve began poring over between meetings at work. And when he gave it a try, a few weeks later, his experience was similar.

Simply put, we both felt better. *Right away.*

Our story probably would have ended with "two middle-aged guys discover cryotherapy works for them," and that would be a pretty boring story, indeed, save for one thing: Both of us saw the retail whole-body cryotherapy experience as something good that could, with a lot of hard work, be turned into something great. Opportunities like that have always inspired us. Indeed, we've been fortunate during our lives, building many successful companies by looking at the way something works and saying, "I can make it work better."

At best, the cryo centers that existed at the time might be described as sterile. At worst, some of them felt like seedy massage parlors. The people running them didn't always know what they were doing; that was nothing short of dangerous. Since a few minutes in a chamber could set someone back a hundred bucks or more, the experience was out of reach for most people. Even folks with plenty of money considered it a once-in-a-while treat, muting the potential therapeutic effects. We opened our first Restore studio determined to fix all those things—and with great confidence that if we did, there would be a long line at the door.

There was. At that door, and the next one, and the next one after that. We're happy to take some credit for those successes, and we're even happier to credit the franchise owners and staff members who have worked so hard to bring this vision to reality. But a big part of Restore's explosive growth comes down to the fact that this was something a lot of people wanted and needed in their lives, and couldn't access before.

If that was true—if cryotherapy had just been sitting there on the sidelines, waiting for someone to figure out how to make it accessible to more people—were there other, similar interventions out there? Ones that both science and people's personal experiences had demonstrated to be effective, but that—for whatever reason—hadn't been widely adopted by the American medical system?

A big part of Restore's explosive growth comes down to the fact that this was something a lot of people wanted and needed in their lives, and couldn't access before.

There were. As our company grew, we added other types of interventions, including hyperbaric oxygen, red light therapy, infrared saunas, therapeutic compression, vitamin-infused IV drips, and intramuscular shots. We had three supreme rules for any therapy we added:

1. Like cryo, each therapy had to have compelling scientific support.
2. Each had to be something most people couldn't access through their personal physician.
3. Each had to be something that helped people feel better right away—because the immediacy of effect was what first sold both of us on the experience of whole-body cryo.

The Virtuous Cycle

All this brings us back to Aldrich Street, to the old guy in the 1970s-style hat, the woman with her high school son, and the cop and the coder and the nurses. The regular crowd. Not athletes eager to mitigate the impacts of aging, as we'd first expected when we began this company, but rather a bunch of regular folks who were a pretty darn good cross-section of our beautifully diverse community.

Oh, we do get plenty of athletes. Our studios and services are used by professional Hall of Famers, active all-stars, Olympic medalists, university champions, blue chip recruits, and top amateurs. It's important to us that people like this—among the healthiest individuals in the world—see value in our services. But that's not our core client because, as it turns out, Restore doesn't have a core client. We've got teenagers and nonagenarians. We've got construction workers and accountants. We've got folks who have come to us as part of their weight-loss journey and others who are working to maintain a lifetime of good fitness. We've got people suffering from arthritis, cancer, migraines, numb nerves, and depression. We've got studios in the trendiest of urban neighborhoods and in a part of the nation better known for being the center of Amish farm country.

We've assembled the experts, we've studied the data, and we've seen the transformations that happen.

One by one, these individuals have affirmed and deepened our belief that right-away interventions aren't just a temporary salve for aches and pains and the symptoms of some ailments. Rather, immediately effective therapies are an essential part of a long-term strategy that can help people slow, stop, and reverse biological aging and chronic diseases.

We do recognize the audacity of that claim. But we've assembled the experts, we've studied the data, and we've seen the transformations that happen when people choose to use these therapies to accentuate immediate wellness and mitigate immediate suffering. These are the starting points for a virtuous cycle—one encapsulated by fourteen words:

When you feel better, you do more. When you do more, you feel better.

A Path for Everyone—Yes, Everyone

The goal of this book is to help you move ever closer to a state of hyper wellness—the point at which a person has reached their full potential of healthfulness, empowering their body to do what it's designed to do, with as little intervention as possible. We'll do a deeper dive on that concept in chapter 1, but for now it suffices to say that wellness is a state in which:

- You are able to exercise your body in meaningful ways, with sufficient recovery that you are able to do so again the next day, and the day after that, and the day after that.
- You rest soundly, getting sleep that recharges your body.
- You eat purposefully, fueling your body with the unique nutrients it needs while still making it fun to eat.
- You nurture your energy, creating capacity to learn new things, challenge your limits, feed your curiosity, expand your boundaries, and offer kindness to yourself.
- You connect deeply with others, building community, acting with decency, giving generously, sharing experiences, being out in the world, and leading with optimism.
- You embrace balance, meeting stress with recovery, aligning work with rest, checking challenge with acceptance, and meeting doing with being.
- You find yourself increasingly able to do more of the things you love.

When you feel better, you do more.
When you do more, you feel better.

In chapter 2, we'll help you identify the aspects of your life that can be seen as obstacles to the goal of hyper wellness, as well as the things you're doing that give you an advantage. These are the mitigatable "headwinds" and augmentable "tailwinds" of wellness, respectively, and it's vital to get a handle on these parts of your life, as they will become the objects of focus for the nine elements of hyper wellness. The elements are a useful framework for thinking about holistic wellness—if you're doing something to impact each of these elements in a positive direction, it's virtually impossible not to be moving toward hyper wellness.

Every therapy we've studied and introduced in Restore studios across the country is aligned to one or more of these elements. It's important to note, though, that none of the practices in this book have to be done at one of our studios. Of course, it would be disingenuous to suggest we *don't* want you to visit a Restore. We do! After all, these places are where we've assembled all these therapies under one roof, with top technologies, expert guidance, and a supportive community of people who are all working toward the goal of hyper wellness. So, if you can make it to one of these locations, this book might be considered a guide to understanding your options, building a personal hyper wellness plan, and getting the most out of each visit. But while our goal is to have a Restore within 20 minutes of virtually every city in the United States in the next few years, we know there are some people for whom a regular visit to one of our studios isn't in the cards. That's fine, because we're also going to help you identify ways to pursue hyper wellness no matter who you are, where you live, how much money you make, how old you are, or what your current state of wellness happens to be. We'll do that in each of the nine chapters aligned to the nine elements—offering you immediately actionable steps you can take to feel better right away. We've put these in an order that makes sense to us, but you don't have to read these chapters in that chronology if you don't want to. Are you curious about cryo? Start there. Are you a lifelong sauna user and want to understand what's happening in your body during long-duration heat exposure? That's a great place to begin. Did you recently listen to a podcast about the health benefits of different kinds of light exposure and want to understand more about how that works? By all means, go directly to that part of the book.

The other way to approach this would be to use the index at the back of the book to identify the challenges you are experiencing and wish to overcome. At the end of this introduction, we have also put together an index of many of the personal health challenges faced and overcome by the dozens of people you will meet in this book, so you can see how these individuals have used the virtuous cycle to attack a problem you might have, too. Many of these folks are our clients but others are not, as we do wish to reiterate this book isn't just for people who happen to live near a Restore studio.

Ultimately, we hope you'll read all the chapters and bring the power of each of these elements into your life. But you're not going to be a passive participant in this journey. You're in the driver's seat.

To that end, once we've described each of the elements—including a review of the evidence that has compelled us to identify and offer related therapies—it will be time for you to decide how to integrate these principles into your life, from the first step you take onto the virtuous cycle to the ultimate goal of hyper wellness. No one can perfectly implement every element of hyper wellness into their lives all at once, after all, and to even try to do so is to invite failure. The journey to hyper wellness is one in which each action reveals the possibilities for the next action, and the actionable possibilities are rapidly expanding in a fast-moving world of health tech research and development. So, in the final chapter, we'll offer you some ideas about how to safely and successfully integrate these principles into your life and how to keep watch for future developments to understand whether they are meritorious or make-believe.

You're not going to be a passive participant in this journey. You're in the driver's seat.

At some point in the process of reading this book, we reckon that you're going to be asking the same question that Steve once did when we were starting down this path together: If all this stuff is so effective, why isn't it *already* part of everyone's health care? Some people think the answer is obvious: There's simply too much money invested in keeping people sick. We're not quite so jaded, but we've seen enough to say that, at the very least, there's not a big rush on the part of the trillion-dollar managed health, health insurance, and pharmaceutical industries to adopt tools and therapies that are intended to accentuate personal wellness.

And what that means is that it's really up to you to take action. We started Restore so that people like you can do just that. And that's also why we've written this book—because we think everyone deserves to be hyper well.

And we believe everyone can be.

Index of Hyper Wellness Success

Acute injury pain
Kaylee, chapter 4

Aging
John, chapter 1
Lanna, chapter 3
Gus, chapter 10
Roy, chapter 10

Alzheimer's disease
Miguel, chapter 8

Anxiety
Larissa, chapter 8

Asthma
Christopher, chapter 9

Athletic performance
Jamal, chapter 5
Keon, chapter 9
Gus, chapter 10
Roy, chapter 10

Atrial fibrillation
Jude, chapter 6

Back pain
John, chapter 1
Tilly, chapter 6
Kris, chapter 12

Chronic pain
Jackie, chapter 3

Cognitive health
Miguel, chapter 8

Depression
Deborah, chapter 2
Anna, chapter 3
Elana, chapter 5
Chhay, chapter 12

Emotional resilience
Marie, chapter 1

Endurance
Jamal, chapter 4

Energy loss
John, chapter 1
Deborah, chapter 2
Nathan, chapter 8
Gina, chapter 9
Chhay, chapter 12

Exercise recovery
Jim, introduction
Steve, introduction
Marie, chapter 1
Shawn, chapter 3
Sergei, chapter 10
Roy, chapter 10

Fatigue
Mitchell, chapter 3
Torben, chapter 4
Christopher, chapter 9

Fibromyalgia
Jackie, chapter 3

Hypohydration
Tilly, chapter 6
Lauren, chapter 6
Tomomi, chapter 6
Jude, chapter 6

Inflammation
Shawn, chapter 3

Injury recovery
Sergei, chapter 10

Involuntary muscle contraction
Rachelle, chapter 3

Joint pain
Marie, chapter 1

Joint stiffness
Marie, chapter 1
Kris, chapter 12

Lack of time
Caishen, chapter 2

Long COVID
Tim, chapter 5
Laurie, chapter 9

Menopause
Macey, chapter 12

Mental fogginess
Mitchell, chapter 3
Jonah, chapter 4
Tomomi, chapter 6

Migraine
Lauren, chapter 6

Mood
Marie, chapter 1
Jonah, chapter 4
Larissa, chapter 8
Ken, chapter 8
Gina, chapter 9

Multiple sclerosis
Rachelle, chapter 3

Muscle pain
Marie, chapter 1

Obesity and weight
Deborah, chapter 2
Peotr, chapter 2
Jude, chapter 6
Gina, chapter 9
Meili, chapter 9
Sergei, chapter 10

Plantar fasciitis
Jennifer, chapter 4

Postpartum fatigue
Erin, chapter 9

Psoriasis
Jonah, chapter 4
Nachelle, chapter 8

Sex drive
Elana, chapter 5

Skin health
Jennifer, chapter 4

Sleep
Parker, chapter 2
Jonah, chapter 4
Jude, chapter 6
Becca, chapter 7
Rob, chapter 7
Payton, chapter 7
Bei, chapter 7
Macey, chapter 12

Sleep apnea
Rob, chapter 7

Stress
Jennifer, chapter 4
Miguel, chapter 8
Ignacio, chapter 9

Ulcerative colitis
Christopher, chapter 9

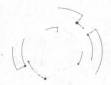

chapter 1

hyper wellness

I t might feel a little silly, but if you're able to get over the initial weirdness of it all, we'd like you to take a journey throughout your entire body. This might be best accomplished while standing in a relaxed position, sitting comfortably in a chair, or lying down, but even if you've got this book propped up on the stand as you're walking on a treadmill, or you're listening to it while driving, you'll still be able to do most of the things we're about to ask you to do.

Let's start with your legs. Everybody's legs are different, of course. Maybe yours aren't quite like the one we'll describe. That's OK. Stick with us as best as you can through this exercise. Begin with your toes. Connect with them, one by one, from the little guy on the end of your left foot to its counterpart on the end of your right foot. Assess each from the tip of the nail to the point where it meets the rest of your foot, and from the tiny phalanges running down the center to the skin wrapped around each digit. Is there an itch? A feeling of warmth? An awkwardness against a crease of your sock? And is there any pain whatsoever, wheresoever? How does all this compare to how your toes could feel, should feel, or have felt in the best moments of your life? Take stock of that perceived difference.

From there, work your way along the bottom of your left foot, the planta pedis, inch by inch, toward your heel, stopping at the flexor digitorum brevis, the muscle right in the middle of the sole. When focused directly on that spot, almost everyone will perceive at least a little bit of soreness; this is a muscle doing a tremendous amount of work with every step you take, after all. Take stock again, then keep moving.

Feel your way around your heel, work back toward your toes, and come up toward your ankle again, this time from the top of your foot, the dorsum. Here is where you're at the best vantage to assess the five metatarsals, the upper outline of which some people can see under their skin when they engage in dorsiflexion, pulling their toes toward their shins. Pause there, head over to your right foot, and repeat what you've just done.

Now you're at your right ankle. Move it around a bit. Feel and listen for a popping sensation as you roll it left, then right, then as you flex outward and as you pull inward. What do you perceive in this large joint, where your heel bone, the talus, meets your tibia and fibula, which run the length of your lower leg?

Keep working up your leg until you get to the knee. This is one of the largest joints in the human body and a spot where many people have their first experience with a major injury—one that takes longer than a few days to heal and often has lasting effects for years or even decades to come. That's because, while our knees are designed to bend, twist, float, and glide,[1] they're inadequate for the ways in which we often use them in the so-called primes of our lives, particularly in the context of the sports we play.[2] As a result, people who have had an injury to this joint in their youth or young adult years can often still feel some residual pain, stiffness, or immobility for the rest of their lives. Are you "carrying around" a problem knee? Take note, then keep moving toward your upper thigh. Work your way, layer by layer, outside to in, from the skin to the fascia to the muscle to the femur, the largest bone in the body, then head back to the left ankle and work your way up that leg as well.

We're just now arriving at the hips and, around back, to the largest muscle of the body, the gluteus maximus, which we exert enormous pressure upon when we sit and which is largely responsible for keeping the trunk of the body upright when we stand. Most people don't really want to contemplate their own butt, but spend some time mindfully assessing this marvelous muscle. Almost everyone carries a little pain or soreness here, or in their gluteus minimus, which is located deeper and extends to the front of the hips, or in their gluteus medius, which rests just above the upper curve of the butt. Do you?

The natural place to go from here might be your body's core, but there's a lot to unpack in there, so instead we'd like you to leave this area and focus on your arms, working your way from your fingers to your shoulders, one side at a time, just as you did with your legs. Once you've done that, you'll be close to your neck—yet another area where many people carry pain and stiffness. Focus on your skin, your muscles, and then your cervical spine—the C1 through C7 vertebrae, and the tissues in between, which are known as the intervertebral discs. Move forward, toward your throat. Swallow softly. Swallow hard. What do you feel?

Now, as we move back to the lower part of your core, we'd like you to feel for discomfort of any sort in your genitals, bowels, and stomach. Is there cramping? Gas? Bloating? Burning? Tenderness? We know how awkward this is, but this is important, so please do spend some time focusing your perceptive attention on all that plumbing down there. When in your life did that part of your being feel *right*? How does it compare to how it feels now?

Now, move up to your chest—to your lungs, esophagus, ribs, and heart. Breathe in as deeply as you can. What do you perceive at the height of that intake of air? Take a few recovery breaths, and then breathe out as much as you can. When you have expelled all the air from your lungs, do you notice a wheeze, a trembling, or a cough?

We're almost done with this exercise, but we still need to tend to our head—a part of the body often and incorrectly considered separate from the rest of our selves, as if part of our being exists below our neck and the other part exists above it. Move your jaw around. Feel for stiffness. Listen for a sound like soft popping or grating sandpaper. Use your tongue to work around the inside of your mouth, looking for spots that are rough or sore on your hard and soft palate and inside gums, then use it to push, one by one, against the inside of each tooth. Tap your teeth together—right side molars, then left side molars, then the incisors and canines in the front. Is anything loose or painful?

Pinch your nose, let go, and then take another deep breath, this time focused on how the air feels as it moves through your nostrils, into the nasal cavity, and past your olfactory nerves. Do you notice any difficulty bringing air into your body in this way? Any congestion? Direct your perception to the sinuses under your cheekbones, the bridge of your nose, and forehead. Roll your eyes around and about. Take a few hard blinks. Are your eyes dry? Is there soreness in any of the thin rectus muscles that surround your eyeball and help it move in all these directions?

Finally, inch by inch, move from the front of your cranium toward the frontal lobe of your brain, around the sides toward your temples, which rest just outside of the temporal lobe, and up from there toward the top of your brain, the parietal lobe, and down toward the back of your skull, which covers the occipital lobe and, just below it toward the back of your neck, the cerebellum. Assess these areas for headache, migraine, tension, throbbing, or clusters of pain. But also take stock of whether you feel clear in thought, alert, awake, and content.

What did you discover?

Waiting for the Unbearable

If you're like everyone else we've known who has gone through an exhaustive, contemplative exploration of your body, you perceived something that, at a bare minimum, is "not quite right." What's more, in most cases, people who engage in this exercise will take note of not one area of concern but dozens of places in their bodies with some level of discomfort and often outright pain. If they do it again in a year, many of those problems will still be there. If they do it again in two years, it will become obvious that not only are these persistent problems, but they are problems that have grown in severity, mostly little by little but sometimes in leaps and bounds.

We've grown so used to these feelings that we usually don't even associate them with deficits in wellness. We say, "I've got a little bit of pain in my foot today," or "that's a strange sensation in my gut—I hope it goes away soon" or "my eyes are just tired right now." And unless these problems acutely prevent us from doing something we need to do, we dismiss them—even if they stick around for a long, long time. At that point it's "oh, well that's just my old trick knee" or "I always have a bit of a headache in that spot" or "my neck is always stiff in the morning."

It's only when these discomforts start to become unbearable that most people even consider seeking help. Indeed, we often dismiss these signs even when we know a symptom could be linked to a deadly disease. Researchers have found half of the people who responded to a survey about early cancer warning signs had experienced an "alarm" symptom, such as an unexplained lump or sudden and unintentional weight loss—and some were aware these symptoms could be related to cancer. Even knowing that, though, many of them declined to contact a doctor about their concerns.[3] Most had decided to sit back, wait, and see if things "got worse." Maybe *then* they'd go see a doctor. Or maybe they'd wait some more. Physicians and researchers have found similar resistance in people with symptoms related to heart disease, diabetes, and a wide range of mental health disorders. This might seem completely illogical, but it's also important to recognize that many people struggle to afford a single visit to a doctor—even with insurance, since most policies have large deductibles to meet before assistance kicks in. Others have felt the sting of having previous concerns dismissed by physicians and don't wish to go through that experience again.

This becomes more alarming when we recognize these are the problems we can perceive. There are many we cannot. Nothing "feels" wrong when a single cell begins to malignantly mutate—and even as a cancer grows and metastasizes, the effects are almost always imperceivable. Often, symptoms come along only when the disease is rampant. Likewise, most people can't perceive the moment in which a gradual accumulation of toxic exposures finally upends the delicate and dynamic chemistry of their blood, setting off a chain reaction of harmful responses as their bodies adjust to maintain metabolism. And as anyone who has ever dealt with a mental health condition (most of us, at one point in our lives) can attest, there is rarely a single, obvious moment in which one's brain shifts from "everything's fine" to "something's wrong." These shifts are gradual and imperceptible at first—which is why so many people wait so long to seek help. It's the proverbial boiling frog.

But it doesn't have to be that way.

Of Math and Morbidity

The way we approach the task of battling injuries, ailments, and diseases has long used disease-level symptoms as the starting place for treatment, such that the term "sick care" is a far more accurate description of modern medicine than the far more common term "health care." If you have any doubts about this, just call a local physician's office and ask for an appointment. Among the first questions they'll ask, of course, is "What are your symptoms?" The expectation is a patient who is *already* perceptibly symptomatic, with the number and severity of those symptoms guiding the process of triage to determine whether someone will be seen right away, next week, next month, next year, or not at all. This is how it works in privatized and socialized medical systems alike.

A lot happens inside our bodies between the time in which we begin to feel "less than our best" and the time in which a physician says, "You need treatment." But it's not just injuries and diseases that are getting worse during this time. It's our holistic state of wellness—our ability to engage in the world at a level commensurate with our interests, aptitudes, and desires.

A lot happens inside our bodies between the time in which we begin to feel "less than our best" and the time in which a physician says, "You need treatment."

This is raw math—not tremendously more complicated than a simple depreciation equation that estimates a reduction in capacity with the passage of time. With each fractional move away from a theoretical "perfect" state of wellness, the deficits compound, and we miss out on a little more of our potential to satiate those interests, engage those aptitudes, and fulfill those desires. But if we improve the rate of change such that capacity *increases*, the whole world changes in the other direction. This is the promise of right-away wellness, and what makes sick care such a tragedy. As a society we've long told people they must wait to feel better, and we've been failing miserably at helping people feel better *right away*, even though that's clearly the most opportune time to intervene.

So, why don't we have health care that intervenes sooner, accenting immediate wellness and alleviating immediate suffering before things get out of hand? In no small part, we can thank a man named Henry Pritchett, who, as president of the Carnegie Foundation for the Advancement of Teaching in the early 1900s, had his fingers on the purse strings of the largest single philanthropic charitable trust ever established at that point in history. Among Pritchett's greatest priorities was the reformation of

American medical schools, and he directed much of the foundation's enormous wealth toward propping up the country's best research-based institutions—those with the capacity to investigate and test treatments for the most pernicious diseases of the day, including pneumonia, flu, tuberculosis, gastrointestinal infections, and smallpox. These investments were hugely successful, and many of the deadliest diseases from a hundred years ago are now treatable conditions, while others have been almost entirely eradicated. The unintended consequence of this focus, however, was that the schools training doctors for most of the 20th century were less focused on holistic wellness. So, even though people could increasingly go to their doctors for life-saving treatment when they became sick, their physicians didn't often have the knowledge, skills, or time to help patients stay well in the first place.

Hospitals in the early 1900s were also struggling to balance their responsibilities to provide life-saving care with the need to stay solvent, particularly as the Great Depression left many patients unable to pay for the care they were receiving. To address this concern at the 400-bed hospital he helped administer in Texas, Baylor University vice president Justin Kimball devised a plan that would allow local teachers to pay 50 cents per month for "prepaid" care. In December 1929, a teacher named Alma Dickson slipped on an icy sidewalk and fractured her ankle. She was hospitalized over Christmas and released without a bill, having become the first person to be served by modern medical insurance.[4] In the coming decades, as both private and socialized systems gained traction around the globe, the insurance model—which paid for care administered after serious problems developed—dictated the ways care was distributed. Insurers became bigger and more powerful. Care became more specialized and more expensive.

But the breaks-before-fixes structure remained. All the while the fundamental depreciation equation that leads small ailments and injuries to whittle away at a person's capacity for hyper wellness continued unabated, and generations of people would never know anything other than sick care.

It's time for us to change this dynamic, first by noting that identifying and mitigating even the smallest deficits in wellness is not an irrational obsession. Rather, this exercise can be best thought of as the starting point for a reimagined kind of insurance in which investments are applied to bolster immediate health, thereby preventing today's discomforts from becoming tomorrow's disabilities, all while providing greater capacity to take other meaningful steps toward hyper wellness.

Identifying and mitigating even the smallest deficits in wellness is not an irrational obsession.

Yes, what we're asking you to do, right now, is to completely upend the way you think about health care. And as long as we're doing that, there's another concept that we'd like you to start thinking differently about: aging.

Age versus Aging

For the first part of the 2021 Myrtle Beach Marathon, Ken Rideout stationed himself behind another runner, just trying to stay out of that morning's ocean breeze. When the winds eased, right around the time they reached mile 16, Rideout made his move—and there wasn't another runner in sight for the rest of the race.

The former prison guard and recovered drug addict finished the 26.2-mile course in just under 2 hours 31 minutes. It was his first marathon victory. It was also the day before his 50th birthday![5]

Fifty is such a fascinating age. Most of us know someone who, at 50, is physically fit in ways we can hardly fathom. They are emotionally poised.

They are as mentally sharp as ever, even more than ever. Whether they are religious or not, they live life with a distinct spiritual serenity, a balance of doing and being. And if someone who didn't know that person's actual age had to guess, based only on appearances, they might guess on the very low side of things.

Most of us also know someone who, at the age of 50, is out of shape, beaten up, tired, and losing steam. They are either psychologically fragile or emotionally unavailable or both. They are mentally degrading. They are spiritually lackluster, unable to mindfully exist in the moment or contemplate anything greater than themselves. And if someone who didn't know them were asked to estimate their age, that guess would be on the high side.

Of course, most folks at any adult age are somewhere between these two extremes. They are physically but not emotionally healthy. Or they are mentally but not spiritually fit. There's a spectrum to all these descriptors.

Where each person falls along that spectrum has long been thought to have been mostly a matter of genetic programming. Some people are destined to age a bit slower, and they're like the first person we envisioned. Other people are designed to experience aging a bit faster, and they're more like the second person.

Each of us can play a big role in the rate at which we experience aging.

There is some truth to this way of thinking about aging, although not as much as many people assume. By following genetically identical twins over time and tracking their outward appearance, rates of disease, and molecular markers of aging, early research on this question suggested that genes account for less than a third of how we age. That meant that about two-thirds of aging was attributable to something else. More recently, though, researchers employing large data sets and models that account for even more factors have concluded that heritability accounts for as little as 7 percent of how a person ages.[6] The other 93 percent is based on a person's environment and, especially, their lifestyle choices, such as what they choose to eat, how they choose to exercise, and whether they choose to smoke. In other words, each of us can play a big role in the rate at which we experience aging. Importantly, this doesn't mean we simply change the fact that we *feel* the effects of aging. It literally means that we can change aging itself.

In mice and other model organisms, scientists have already demonstrated the ability to slow down and even reverse the symptoms of aging—from graying hair and wrinkled skin to weakening muscles and thinning blood vessels—using drugs and supplements aimed at restoring the energy-transporting molecules that are lost in nearly all animals as they experience aging. Although it will still be some time before any of these interventions could potentially be approved by regulating bodies like the US Food and Drug Administration and the European Medicines Agency, which are the standard-bearers for safety and efficacy of medical treatments and therapies, many people are already seeking to implement these treatments in their lives. Others have been more cautious—which is an understandable approach, given the many questions that have not yet been resolved about how and whether these interventions work in human beings. But the vast majority of people are not in either of the "go for it" or "wait and see" camps, because they are still living under the assumption that aging inexorably comes with age.

Before anyone can make progress toward understanding their own wellness, let alone hyper wellness, they must be able to decouple these concepts. So, let's do that: Age is *not* aging.

Age is a unit of time. One voyage around the sun. Two voyages. And so on. This rate is fixed. There's nothing we can do about it.

Aging, on the other hand, comprises the progressive physiological changes that lead to a decline of physical and mental function. This does not happen universally to our entire bodies but rather emerges unevenly across each of our biological systems and subsystems, and even across each of the 37 trillion cells of our bodies.

When we are young and healthy, almost all our cells function very effectively. Over time, though, our cells begin to break down, and the organs and systems they are part of eventually stop working. The result is less energy and more pain, the earliest signs of holistic aging, which can be thought of as being inversely proportional to holistic wellness. As aging increases, wellness decreases; as wellness improves, aging is mitigated.

This is vital to understand, not only because extreme aging is so brutal, but because aging invites disease. There is no factor that is a greater predictor of heart disease, cancer, stroke, diabetes, and dementia than aging. So, when we slow aging, we also slow all these diseases—a double benefit that results in longer healthspans, the period of life lived without aging-related diseases or disabilities.

To be clear, neither of us is an immortalist; we both believe that everyone will die eventually. We are also not enamored with the view that healthy lifespan extension, in the extreme, is a categorically good idea, even if it was possible. Some very credible scientists have suggested that it's reasonable to assume that healthspans of 120 years and longer may become common in the future,[7] but as a society we would need to make some revolutionary changes to keep that sort of future from being a dystopian one. But while this idea shouldn't be dismissed as fanciful, most people are still many, many decades from anything close to that sort of longevity.

In the meantime, however, what the current research suggests is that even if all medical progress ended at this very moment—if we could rely only on the treatments and therapies we have today—we would still have everything we need to secure 16 to 25 additional years of healthy life for just about anyone. That's possible simply by making lifestyle choices that result in a slowing of aging—or, in the inverse way of thinking, an increase in wellness.

Let's just consider that more conservative number—16 years—and remember, as we do, that we are not simply talking about more years but more *healthy* years: Who would not want to spend an extra decade and a half living, loving, learning, and giving? Who would not want to get to see their grandchildren and great-grandchildren grow and thrive?

Now, let's be even more optimistic (as we both are). Who would not want all that for another quarter-century—or perhaps even longer?

We do. Do you? If so, hyper wellness is the path.

Setting a Hyper Wellness Trajectory

There is one important caveat to the view of wellness and aging as inversely proportional concepts: The years we've lived, the stresses we've faced, and the decisions we've made cannot be undone, and thus, as Shakespeare wrote in one of his most famous works, "Things without all remedy should be without regard." There is no sense feeling guilty for that which has resulted in our current state of wellness. Lady Macbeth was right: "What's done is done." Some of the consequences of those years, stresses, and decisions may not be undone, and so we must come to the goal of hyper wellness with a realistic expectation of potential—albeit an expectation that, as you will see, is often far greater than most people initially allow themselves to believe.

That was the surprise awaiting John, a client at the first studio we opened in Austin. John had suffered a back injury when he fell off a roof at the age of 25 and carried significant pain in his spine ever since. We met him in his early 60s, a time in which he was additionally experiencing a slow decline in energy during and after his biweekly workouts. That's not unusual with aging, and it's what first brought John into our studio for cryotherapy, which has long been associated with decreases in fatigue during exercise.[8]

John's experiences with cryo came with an increase in energy—which is what he was hoping for—but it also led to a substantial decrease in the pain in his back, an experience also aligned to research findings[9] but one that John hadn't so much as dreamed of experiencing himself.

"I've got to say that was a shock," he told us. "I felt like I'd tried everything over the years, but it just kept getting worse. That pain was part of me. It was always there. And I can't say that now, with cryo, it's like I was never injured at all, but there are lots of times now when I don't notice the pain."

But John also figures he hasn't reached his full potential. And, in fact, he can't, for there is no "perfect" state of hyper wellness. There's always room for growth toward potential. And that's an important part of the process. By continuously working toward the goal of bringing his lived experience closer to potential, staying on the virtuous cycle, John is working against the sorts of "small slides" away from wellness that—little by little, and especially for people who are of a greater age—lead to aging and disease.

Thus, one of the most vital steps toward hyper wellness is an assessment of potential. How do we ascertain what is immutable versus what can actually be improved? Here's a good rule-of-thumb question: Have others in similar circumstances experienced improvement?

It might seem hard to believe that every malady that someone else has mitigated is a problem that you can fix as well, and you might not be the kind of person who can embrace that level of optimism, or who isn't ready to do so just yet. That's fine and reasonable. You don't need to believe that you can reach the *apex* of your wellness potential in order to begin moving in that direction. But it's important to understand what is possible, even if those possibilities seem like they could only exist in the extreme, for this is what allows us to take a first step knowing that if and when that step proves successful, it won't be the last. Thus we keep moving, we keep improving, we keep growing, and we keep healing. We get closer and closer to becoming hyper well.

You don't need to believe that you can reach the apex *of your wellness potential in order to begin moving in that direction.*

Taking a Wellness Census

No perceptible improvement in wellness is too small to matter, for capacity is cumulative. If we have many problems to address—as most people do—it also doesn't matter what specific problem is solved first, because a boost in any one part of our wellness will make the next improvement more likely. So, while it makes sense to target a precise problem, it's not necessarily a failure if the first intervention we try doesn't mitigate that specific issue, particularly if we perceive a benefit in some *other* area of our life.

This will become clearer as we dive into many of the therapies we will discuss in this book. None of these interventions are targeted at just one problem; the research tells us that all of them can be multidimensionally effective. By way of example, we'd like to introduce you to Marie, who at the age of 53 decided to become intentional about addressing a problem she had been dealing with for many years, chronic joint pain, which was preventing her from exercising.

Marie hadn't heard about whole-body cryotherapy at that time, but she had heard that ice baths could be effective for reducing joint pain. So, every evening before she worked out, Marie would fill a bathtub with cold water and drop in as many ice cubes as she was able to make in her freezer that day. She would slide into the tub, staying immersed in the frigid water as long as she could, and then get out. She did this for a week, then two, hoping she would be among the group of people for whom this therapy works to alleviate joint pain.

As it turned out, her joints *didn't* feel any better. They didn't feel worse, but there was no perceptible improvement in this aspect of her wellness. It was still painful to exercise.

What Marie did notice, however, was a perceptible change in mood. "It wasn't a huge difference, at first, but it was noticeable," she said. "I was waking up less unhappy and more content."

This makes plenty of sense, because research has shown that even a single session of cold-water immersion can lead to significant emotional boost.[10]

There is a wealth of clinical evidence showing that exercise can improve one's mood, but the opposite is also true: When our emotional states improve, we have more resilience. We can exercise more. So, Marie did. She was still feeling pain and stiffness in her joints. But she had the emotional capacity to go just a little bit farther in the face of those challenges. Instead of looking sadly at the exercise bike in her living room and deciding she just couldn't do it, she would hop on and pedal for a few minutes. And no, this wasn't the Ironman Triathlon, but it was a little bit more than she could do before, and after a few weeks she found she could do even more. The *targeted* problem hadn't subsided, but Marie was nonetheless deriving a wellness benefit. That's a meaningful success. Yet if Marie looked at this experience only through the lens of whether it improved her joint pain, she would have seen it as a failure.

We do tend to miss things we are not looking for, and there are few better examples of this than the famous "invisible gorilla" experiment, which employs a video of six people—three of them wearing white shirts and three wearing black—who are moving about and passing basketballs with one another. People watching the video are asked to count the passes made by the individuals wearing white. Most people who watch the video get the right answer of passes, or come close, but what many viewers also miss is that, in the middle of the video, a person wearing a gorilla costume strolls into the middle of the passing circle, thumps its chest, and then walks away. If you watch the video and know to look for the gorilla, you can't miss it. But if you don't, it's astounding how easy it is to not even notice the person in the ape suit.

We do tend to miss things we are not looking for.

This is why a "wellness census" is so important, preferably (but not mandatorily) before you engage in any of the therapies we will be detailing later in this book. There are many different ways to conduct such an assessment, but perhaps the easiest starting point is to take a journey through your body, much like the exercise we suggested at the start of this chapter. When you move methodically throughout your body, you'll come to recognize the places that are not doing what they are designed to do, in either obvious ways or more subtle ways. When we earlier described this whole-body assessment, we suggested you make a mental note of those issues, but when you go through this process again it would be beneficial to first turn on an audio recorder. You might not have a medically proper name for what you discover, and that's OK. The truth is that there might not *be* a clinical definition for what you're feeling. So just do your best to describe it. You might simply say something like "There's a warm, slightly painful feeling under my left shoulder" or "There's a faint pinching sensation below my ribs when I take a deep breath."

Do this with your body at rest. Do it again as you stretch in every direction you can manage, and then again with your body in motion at a slow and comfortable pace of walking, and again at a jog, and then again at whatever speed of running, swimming, biking, or other cardiovascular exercise you can maintain at length, making verbal notes along the way. It might be a good idea to do this several times over a week or two, then transcribe your audio notes into a document or, better yet, a spreadsheet.

A medical exam is a wise second step, as your physician may recognize problems that you do not. A slight heart murmur. Blood pressure a little on the high side of a healthy range. A bit of damage in your ear canal.

Many well-intentioned doctors won't even make note of issues that they feel are "typical" for someone of your age, so it's important to let your physician know that you'd like them to alert you to *anything* that could be improved, even if they don't view it as an area of great concern. Add your doctor's observations to your list.

Physical exams are often accompanied by a few routine tests, including a blood panel. Most patients never look at the results of these tests—they rely on their doctors to tell them if anything is wrong. But many physicians are reluctant to flag anything that isn't far away from the putatively healthy "reference range" of upper and lower limits, so it's good to see these numbers with your own eyes. If you can't access a blood panel from your physician, consider getting a test done in a private clinic, at a studio like Restore, or from a reputable online testing provider. Don't panic over what you see when your data arrives. Don't seek to diagnose yourself. Just become aware of these data, and add the numbers to your list.

We shouldn't neglect mental health. Just about everyone can benefit from a formal psychological assessment, but if you're feeling mentally fit, there's not necessarily a pressing reason to take on that burden of time and expense. What can be helpful over the long term, however, is one of the many self-assessments that are available online and are backed by a reputable clinical source, preferably one that allows you to provide your answers on a scale and to see and save those answers over time. If taking a test like this alerts you to a potential struggle that you might need some help addressing, that's a positive outcome. But even if no substantial problems are revealed through a self-assessment, it's good to remember that more than 50 percent of people will be diagnosed with a mental health disorder at some point in their life, so keeping this data as a baseline may be valuable down the road.

There are ways to go much deeper—and depending on your time, interest, and resources, this can be advantageous. Your personal genetic code won't ever change, but many people find it beneficial to undergo personal

DNA sequencing, especially as research has made it increasingly possible to connect specific genes, and combinations of genes, to one's risks for many health conditions. This can be done via mail through reputable companies, but some people who are worried that they might mess up the process if they do it themselves prefer to have it done at a testing lab in their community.

In contrast to your unchanging genetic code, your epigenome—a collection of molecular markers that rest on everyone's DNA and have the power to modulate genetic expression—is malleable over time, and is increasingly being connected to propensities for physical and mental wellness. The epigenome may also be the best place to assess biological aging. Tests that measure various epigenetic markers, including those that are associated with aging, are increasingly accessible and affordable.

Finally, there are a growing number of biomarkers that aren't often part of the routine clinical testing most people get from their physicians, but that have been demonstrated to be useful, particularly in association with the ways in which our bodies utilize nourishment. Knowing this data can help you see changes when and if they come, which is why biomarker testing has been among the most sought-after services we offer at Restore.

People will go about all this in different ways. Some will want to have as many data points as possible to assess and track their wellness over time. Others get overwhelmed by stuff like this; for them, a simple self-assessment of how their body feels will be enough. Most folks will be somewhere in the middle as a condition of interest, time, and resources. There is no right answer. Do what you can and what feels right for you.

If you don't do anything, though, it's almost certain you're going to miss the gorilla in the middle of the room. And while that doesn't render the process toward hyper wellness impossible, it will slow down the journey.

Not sure how you feel about this one way or another? Start small. Make a ranked list of 10 things you're already aware of that you'd like to improve upon, and target the top item on that list, while keeping watch for changes to the others. Over time you may decide to be more regimented, and that's fine, too. The important takeaway is that you put yourself in a position to perceive improvements in your wellness—the "feel better" part of the virtuous cycle—because that's when the "do more" part comes into play.

There is no right answer. Do what you can and what feels right for you.

Getting to the First Rotation

Once you've done *something* and felt better because of it, it's time to do *something else.* If the first therapy you tried addressed the problem you were targeting in sufficient measure that it's no longer a problem, then it's obvious that you'll need to select another target. Consult the document you created as a result of your wellness census, identify an issue that has potential for mitigation, find the research-backed interventions that have been demonstrated to be effective (this book will hopefully be a great resource for you in this regard, but we encourage you to become comfortable searching the vast library of peer-reviewed literature available from the National Center for Biotechnology Information), and get to it.

What might not be so obvious, however, is what to do if the therapy you tried didn't sufficiently address the problem you were targeting. At first blush, it might seem that the right answer would be to choose another intervention that research suggests may positively impact that same area of concern, but that may or may not be the right approach at this point in your journey toward hyper wellness.

Here's why: People often try to alleviate the biggest problem they are facing. And this makes some sense, because eliminating big problems can pay big dividends in terms of capacity: If you're successful, you'll feel *a lot* better. Ergo, you'll be able to do *a lot* more. The virtuous cycle will start with a turbo-charged success!

But big problems generally become big problems because they are akin to an extensive quantity—a principle from classical mechanics that describes a system whose magnitude is the sum of its subsystems, and that can be applied to biological systems as well. So, if a therapy documented to often have a beneficial effect doesn't result in that intended effect, the reason might be because the complexity of the problem outweighs the directness of the solution.

Or, at least, that might be the case *at this moment*—but it doesn't mean that all hope for mitigation is lost. Rather, it means that the best approach may be to move on to another target, seeking to build capacity a little at a time for an eventual run at that bigger, more extensive problem.

For instance, the first issue Marie identified for intervention was stiffness in her joints. The nightly ice baths didn't at first seem to be having any success in addressing that issue, but she did seem to be in a better mood, and that provided her with a bit of energy for more exercise. The truth is that there are a lot of other interventions for sore joints that have a good deal of research to back their effectiveness. Heat can help,[11] as can acupuncture.[12] So can meditation,[13] massage,[14] and some supplements.[15]

But joint pain wasn't the *only* problem Marie was facing. She also retained soreness in her muscles for days after she exercised. That was never a big problem—it's something that many people deal with as they experience aging—but now that she was exercising a little bit more, the soreness seemed to be sticking around a little bit longer. Although this was never the most pressing problem on her list, it was an issue with a lot of demonstrated potential for mitigation—particularly through compression therapy.[16] When Marie learned this, she purchased a set of compression tights, and she made a habit of putting them on right after her post-workout shower. Soon, she noticed a subtle change: The muscle pain she was experiencing wasn't lasting as long as it did before! And so she could exercise a bit more often.

This is what we call a "rotation" on the virtuous cycle—the moment in which an intervention leads to an improvement that, in turn, permits you to engage in another intervention. Marie tried an intervention, it helped her feel better, so she could do more. She tried another, and it also helped her feel better, and now she could do more again. And the awesome thing that happened, in her case, is that these two interventions were working in tandem to permit more exercise—which is itself an intervention that accentuates wellness and slows aging.[17]

Is this the point at which a person's joint pain begins to be alleviated? For some people, perhaps. Exercise has repeatedly been shown to be effective for this problem.[18] For Marie, it would take a few more rotations of the cycle, but we are happy to report that she did eventually arrive at a life of substantially reduced pain and increased mobility!

No one is like anyone else. We all have different challenges and different goals. We're also all going to choose different therapies, based on what is available and affordable—or perhaps based on what seems most intriguing to us as individuals. Some people see a cryotherapy chamber and think, "Hell yeah!" Others see one of these machines and say, "Oh my, I'm not sure about that." That therapy might work on both types of people, but if someone is initially nervous or skeptical about an intervention, that's probably not the right starting place for them, and it might not ever be something they're willing and able to try. There's nothing wrong with that. We're all going to take a different path toward hyper wellness.

What is important for everyone, equally, is *staying on* the virtuous cycle—using a little bit of the capacity you earn with each rotation to do more, so that you can continue to make progress toward your potential.

We're all going to take a different path toward hyper wellness.

Live More

As we mentioned, research suggests that in the long term, the virtuous cycle we've described may accentuate wellness and slow aging enough to offer 16 to 25 additional years of healthy life. But while good health can help promote happiness, these words are not synonymous. Indeed, over the years most of us have met some people who appear to be fit and vigorous well into their 80s and 90s, and yet they don't appear to be happy. They're cantankerous. They're miserly. They don't seem to have many close friends or devoted family members. It's sad.

If we're not using the healthy years we earn by virtue of a hyper wellness lifestyle to do the things that bring joy to our lives, then what's the point?

The same can be said for the short term. The capacity you generate as a result of therapies that prove successful for alleviating immediate suffering and accentuating immediate health can be wholly turned toward "doing more" in terms of more such interventions. This is just what smart novice entrepreneurs do when they first turn a profit. They don't buy a fancy new car; instead, they reinvest in their business. In the same way, it can be good to reinvest all your earned capacity into your immediate health when you are only a few rotations into your journey toward hyper wellness. This itself can be a source of joy for many people. But if you don't *ultimately* use some of this capacity to bring joy to your life in other ways, then, again, what's the point?

If you've been suffering from joint pain, and your path toward hyper wellness has alleviated that pain enough so that you can exercise more, then by all means use that capacity to exercise more. But also use it to go on walks with your friends. Use it to play a sport with your children or grandchildren. Use it to take up a new hobby. Use it to volunteer to help people in need in your community. Use it to bring joy to your life—right now. Use it to feel alive, fulfilled, loved, needed, and purposeful. Wonderfully, investing in yourself in these ways is capacity-generating, too, for when we live a life of joy, we want it to keep going, thus we generate fuel for the next turn of the virtuous cycle, and the next after that, and the next after that.

Along the way, you'll hit some obstacles—many that will reveal themselves early into this journey, and some that will appear only once the voyage is well underway. But you'll also soon recognize that there are elements of your life that will keep you moving in the right direction, and some of these things are also going to reveal themselves early in this process, while others will come along when you least expect it. These are the "headwinds" and "tailwinds" of the hyper wellness lifestyle, and before we begin a deep exploration of how to mitigate and accentuate these winds, we need to know where to find them.

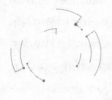

chapter 2

headwinds and tailwinds

I t happened so gradually that Deborah almost didn't notice.

The nearly limitless energy she always felt as an athletic teenager had begun to wane in her 20s, but with an intense focus on school and the first few years of her career, she missed this early warning sign that she was slipping away from a state of hyper wellness.

There may have still been time for Deborah to make major changes as she moved into her 30s, but by that time she was focused on her career and family, with three busy children. And even though she knew this was a time that she could make meaningful changes that would impact her for the rest of her life, including a better diet and more exercise, she often felt as though those steps were investments that simply couldn't be made at the time.

"Dinner was always something like drive-through tacos between basketball and ballet and debate team competitions," she recalled. "I told myself the steps I was putting in up the stairs at my kids' schools, or the walks to and from the soccer fields during a tournament, were forms of exercise, even though I knew that wasn't true. It wasn't close to the amount of exercise I actually needed."

With each passing day it seemed as though she was waking up a little more tired than she had been the day before. And in a real way, that was true. By the time Deborah hit 40, the biochemical changes that conspire to lock in a low-energy existence had begun in earnest, and they were progressing quickly. Now, the diet and exercise changes she needed were becoming harder. She was eating high-calorie foods just to get from sunrise to sunset, and didn't feel as though she had enough energy at the end of the day to exercise.

Things got even worse when she tore her anterior cruciate ligament after missing a step on the bleachers at her son's soccer game. For almost a year, exercise felt downright impossible, and while her knee eventually healed following surgery, by that time she had put on 20 pounds.

Researchers have found that weight gain is associated with more time being ill, especially for women,[1] and Deborah attested that she found herself more sick, more often, setting her back at work and leaving her less time to focus on the things she knew could help her maintain her wellness.

"It felt like one more thing would go wrong every year or so, and it all just compounded," she said. "And it got to the point that I felt hopeless and figured this was the way things would keep going for the rest of my life."

Deborah's experience was not at all unusual. We've heard hundreds of stories like hers—cases in which energy loss leads to injury, injury leads to pain, pain leads to weight gain, weight gain leads to illness, and on it goes.

These are some of the "headwinds" that conspire to keep us from any sort of wellness, let alone hyper wellness. But before we dive deeper into these obstacles, we think it's important that you know that Deborah's story has a happy ending—or perhaps we should say it has a "happy middle," because it sure isn't over yet. She's doing great—and we'll get back to that part of the story soon.

First, though, we do need to talk about the most common headwinds we've seen during our years of helping people get on a virtuous cycle, because these are some of the obstacles you may be facing as well.

Energy loss leads to injury, injury leads to pain, pain leads to weight gain, weight gain leads to illness, and on it goes.

Energy Loss

The first and most predictable headwind is energy loss—the same experience Deborah had starting in her 20s—a result of the lapse of mitochondrial function during aging.[2] Mitochondria are often viewed as the "powerhouse" of our cells, but they are also part of the signaling network that helps our cells know how to react to all sorts of stimuli, regulators of immunity when we are confronted with malicious bacteria and viruses, and modulators of stem cell activity across the span of our lives. All of us go through some degree of mitochondrial disfunction as we grow older, and this may itself cause disease,[3] but it definitely causes energy loss.

This link has been most closely studied in skeletal muscle, which connects bones to other bones, thus permitting most voluntary movement.[4] Since skeletal muscle also comprises about a third of most people's body mass, declines in mitochondrial activity in this part of our bodies likely have a significant effect on all aspects of our lives. So while many people have been led to believe that aging-related decline of muscle mass—which generally occurs at a rate of 3 to 8 percent per decade after the age of 30 and tends to accelerate after the age of 60[5]—is a result of less physical activity, the truth is that mitochondria are playing a huge role in this decline.

Thankfully, there is a seemingly simple way to slow mitochondrial exhaustion. "Perhaps the best intervention to counteract this age-dependent decline in muscle function, termed sarcopenia, is physical exercise," Ohio State University biologist Nuo Sun and his colleagues wrote in 2016.[6] But therein lies the rub: We can't exercise without energy! The solution is also the problem! It's a vicious cycle.

In the coming chapters, we're going to spend a lot of time discussing ways in which therapies that offer right-away benefits can counteract that cycle. But we've found that it's often best to just get all the bad news out there at once. So, before we get to those solutions, let's identify some other common headwinds.

Nutrient Absorption

We tend to associate certain foods with certain nutrients. Bananas for potassium. Oranges for vitamin C. Dairy products for calcium. And on it goes. That's not incorrect, but what many people miss is that the ways in which our individual bodies absorb nutrients from foods vary from person to person. It depends on biological sex, genetic background, and lifestyle. It depends on the recency of exercise, the kinds of foods and drinks we've recently consumed, and the level of stress we're experiencing. And perhaps most powerfully of all, it depends on the level at which we have experienced aging. Indeed, even the kinds of foods we generally consider to be the most natural and the healthiest for us are absorbed by our bodies less efficiently when wellness declines.

As we experience aging, it gets harder to acquire the nutrients we need.

It's not hard to see how this can be a powerful headwind working against those who are seeking a greater degree of hyper wellness. Proper nutrition is, after all, at the heart of healthfulness. Yet, as we experience aging, it gets harder to acquire the nutrients we need via food, and even supplementation is hampered by waning efficiency over time. Thus, as we age, we can't just eat and supplement as we always have. We have to eat better. We have to supplement smarter. And if that sounds hard, it's because it certainly can be for many people.

Once again, we want to assure you there are ways to fight back against this headwind. We'll get to those approaches in coming chapters. But, alas, we're not done talking about all the forces that conspire to keep us from achieving wellness.

Disease and Pain

For a long time, many people assumed that cancer was a matter of "the odds catching up to us." Over time, DNA damage accumulates, causing cells to mutate. The more time, the more mutations. The more mutations, the more likely a malignant and transmissible change will occur. And that, in a nutshell, was why the risk of cancer was thought to increase as people become older. In this way of thinking, it was chronological age, not biological aging, that put us most at risk. This was a tidy hypothesis—but recent research has shown that it's incomplete.

In 2017, a study led by Jun Li, then at Harvard Medical School, set the stage for a new view of why older people tend to have an increased risk of cancer. Li and her colleagues reported that cellular repair is greatly affected by levels of nicotinamide adenine dinucleotide, also known as NAD+, an essential regulator of signaling pathways that researchers have long known to be one of the many substances in our bodies that declines with age. As NAD+ decreases with age, the role it serves in regulating the levels of other DNA-repairing molecules is weakened.[7] Thus, the problem is not simply the accumulation of "bad cells" over time; it's also—and perhaps more so—that our bodies become less effective at repairing DNA when it goes awry.

So, in addition to the fact that we tend to lose energy and get less efficient at absorbing nutrients during aging, we also tend to suffer from increasingly ineffective cellular repair—which helps explain not only why cancer rates increase with aging but also why the rates of other diseases increase as well. This also informs our understanding of why it takes longer to heal from injuries, leading to chronic pain. Simply put, our bodies are less able to engage in the repair it takes to remain well, let alone move toward hyper wellness.

That's a tremendous headwind, for disease begets disease. For instance, people with type 2 diabetes, which is mainly lifestyle-related and accumulates over time, are far more likely to suffer from heart disease, stroke, high blood pressure, and atherosclerosis. That's partially because people whose lifestyles lead to diabetes tend to be less healthy in the first place, but it's also because no disease happens in a void. The human body's biochemical response to diabetes can come at the expense of other balances, especially immunological functions that keep other diseases at bay.[8] Couple that with a reduced ability for cellular repair, and you've got the makings of a headwind from hell.

Making matters worse, pain also begets pain, pain sometimes begets disease, and disease often begets pain. You probably already know this to be true—either from your own experience or from the experience of someone close to you.

If you've ever suffered a bad injury to your foot or lower leg, for instance, you might have noticed that at as result of trying to protect the injury during the process of healing, the imbalance in the way you move results in pain somewhere else—often higher up on that same leg, in your hip, or in the lower back or even the opposite leg, which is now doing more of the work as you walk. Maddeningly, this associated pain can sometimes last even longer than the pain from the original injury.

Pain is also a common problem for cancer survivors, especially in the years immediately following remission, and as many as 1 in 10 cancer survivors will end up suffering from long-term pain so severe that it interferes with their ability to enjoy life.[9] The cancer may be gone, but the pain remains.

Pain also compounds. Many golfers know this all too well. Two of the most common injuries for golfers are tendinitis in the elbow and damage to the rotator cuff, the muscles and tendons around the shoulder joint. An elbow injury may come one season. Steady damages to the rotator cuff may accumulate over time and become painful many seasons later. Unfortunately, it's not uncommon for separate areas of pain to merge, resulting in severe discomfort and immobility in a golfer's entire arm. These are the kinds of injuries many of us would have bounced back from earlier in our lives but, as we experience aging and diminished cellular repair, that's no longer the case. And even if there is a potential solution, it often seems like there's a lack of time to fully engage in it.[10]

Time

For a few moments, think back to the major milestones of your life—the moments that have brought you immense joy. For many people, marriage and parenthood are some of the top events on this list. For others, it might be the achievement of an academic degree or a big promotion at work or the purchase of a home they've fallen in love with.

At first, it might sound crazy, and even contemptible, to think of these milestones as headwinds, but the truth is that these moments in life almost always come with added responsibilities, which often means less free time, which often means less sleep, which often means less energy.

Please don't get us wrong: We're not saying that things like finding a partner, having children, succeeding at work, earning a degree, or buying a home should be avoided. As we'll soon see, these are also parts of our lives that can be powerful tailwinds—propelling us forward in our journey toward hyper wellness. But time is finite, and when we find ourselves with less of it to spare, we begin making tradeoffs—just like Deborah did. As she grew older, had more responsibility at work, and dedicated more of her time to her children, she was often choosing between healthy activities and time. When confronted with the choice of healthier home-cooked meals, which take time and energy to prepare, or grabbing fast food, which at least *feels* quicker and easier, she chose the option that she perceived to give her more time. These perceptions are often a mirage, but Deborah's decisions are common. We've all fallen into these sorts of traps at one time or another, and it's virtually incontestable that people with fewer means generally have even less time than those who are more economically fortunate.

One of the people we greatly respect on matters of health has acknowledged this hard truth as well. "It would be delusional of me to say that a single working mom with five kids in the inner city has the same amount of time that the wealthy mom in Beverly Hills has," the physician, podcaster, and author Peter Attia said in 2023. "Of course not. Unfortunately, the truth of it is that health is not fully democratized. There's a certain income level and disposable time requirement that's probably necessary. You don't have to be wealthy, but you have to be above a certain threshold in terms of disposable time and income."[11]

We're not able to upend a social economic structure of haves and have nots, but what we can do is provide people with the tools and knowledge to step on to the virtuous cycle no matter how little time and economic resources they have. Indeed, this is one of the beautiful things about a feel-better-do-more approach to life: The initial investment is so small that anyone can do it, and the expanded capacity created in the process grows from there—no further principal must be invested.

This is one of the beautiful things about a feel-better-do-more approach to life: The initial investment is so small that anyone can do it.

Many people will tell you that willpower is the only thing you need to get started on—and remain on—a journey to better wellness. We are inclined to agree; we're big proponents of bootstraps and not huge fans of excuses. But we're also objectively minded people, and the truth is that individuals who have more time and flexibility in their lives are better able to tap into and utilize both intrinsic and acquired resilience and resolve, the fundamental elements that make willpower possible. Thus, as we focus in later chapters on the strategies most likely to result in improved wellness, we'll discuss ways to build up your reservoir of willpower, but we'll talk a whole lot more about why the effective management and use of time can pay enormous dividends when it comes to hyper wellness.

What Are Your Headwinds?

You've likely recognized one or two or even all of these headwinds in your own life. It's also possible that you haven't yet experienced any of these obstacles to wellness. You haven't felt any loss of energy. Your body is processing nutrients as well as it ever has. You're free of disease and recover quickly from injuries. You don't feel at a loss of time. But even if that's all true, there may still be headwinds in your life that are conspiring to keep you from hyper wellness, and identifying these challenges is an important part of this process.

The essential questions to ask are: What are the things I could be doing to be healthier and happier? And what is keeping me from doing those things?

As you might suspect, the answers to those questions are going to change over time for people who embrace a feel-better-do-more lifestyle. Many of the things that you might not even imagine to be possible in terms of health and happiness today may not look the same after a few turns of the virtuous cycle.

That was the case for Deborah. When she began her journey toward hyper wellness, Deborah couldn't have imagined being able to one day compete in a triathlon. Her headwinds were too strong. She didn't have the energy. She didn't have the time. She wasn't getting the full nutritional benefit of the foods she was eating. Her body wasn't healing as fast as it once did. Although she had always loved swimming and biking, had competed in cross-country in high school, and had friends who had competed in triathlons before, that sort of thing wasn't even on her radar.

So, the first time she asked herself about the things she could be doing to be healthier and happier, being able to run one mile, without stopping, was as far as she could dream. "And even then," she said, "that was a really big dream—something I wasn't sure I could ever actually do."

The next question she had to ask was what was keeping her from even attempting that goal, and she quickly identified nearly all the headwinds we've already discussed. But Deborah also recognized some others, and the one that seemed it might be the hardest to overcome was the depression she had been experiencing since her 20s.

"I don't think my mental health was anything close to as bad as what some people deal with, but it was always a problem," she said. "I had to do things like go to work and drive my kids to school, but I never felt like I wanted to do any of those things, so I think I was expending a lot of energy just getting myself to do the things I really had to do to stay employed and be a good mom. Now, when I look back on those years, I can see that I didn't have much energy for anything that I knew could be put off. And exercise could always be put off."

When a friend who had also fought depression told Deborah that she had perceived a significant change in her mood since starting a monthly routine of getting an intravenous drip of NAD+, Deborah was skeptical. There have been some early studies indicating that NAD+ supplementation could be a promising treatment for depressive behaviors,[12] and more research is underway, but most of the evidence of its effectiveness for this health challenge is still anecdotal. Still, Deborah was willing to give it a try.

To be clear: The IV drip didn't "cure" Deborah's depression. "I guess the best way to describe it is that it seemed to take the edge off," she said. "I went from a baseline of sort of trudging through things to feeling like I had a little more energy for the things I had to do, and I think that left a little more in the tank for the things I wanted to do, like trying to run again."

It was hard at first. She could barely jog a quarter mile around the track at the local high school, and she wasn't fast. But she gradually gained endurance and, eventually, she reached her goal: She could run a mile without stopping. In fact, she could do it day after day.

That's when she was able to again ask herself about other things she could be doing to be healthier and happier. "And that's when I had this absurd thought in my head that a triathlon was something that was possible," she said.

The biggest headwind that would make that goal difficult was time. Training for a tri is a big commitment even for those who are very fit. Deborah was getting fitter by the day, but she still had a long way to go. In consultation with a triathlon coach, she figured she would need about 15 hours a week just for training. But having sustained one headwind, she felt more confident that she could overcome another.

Part of that process was sitting down with her children and asking them to help support her—riding their bikes to school, arranging to share rides whenever possible, and picking up a few more responsibilities around the house. "I cry a little every time I think about that conversation," she said (and indeed, at this point in our conversation she did begin tearing up). "They didn't flinch. They didn't complain. And they didn't just commit to doing the things I asked—they came up with other ways to help make sure I'd have time to train." The next morning, for instance, Deborah's oldest son woke up early to make breakfast for his siblings and mom—a habit he continued every day for the next year.

Deborah didn't complete her first triathlon. She finished the swim and the ride but fell out during the transition to the run. But she didn't give up, either, and the last time we checked in with her she had competed in five of these races—and completed four of them!

You might have noticed that Deborah didn't succeed in this way simply because she was able to identify and mitigate many of her headwinds. She also had the love and support of her family, something that had been there all along—the very sort of available but often underutilized forces that we have come to think of as tailwinds.

Initiating and Secondary Tailwinds

The physical laws of the universe dictate every element of our lives. From the atoms that make up everything in the immediate world around us to the trillions of galaxies in our known universe, *everything* is either growing or decaying.

That includes our health. At every moment of our life, we are moving either toward wellness or toward aging. Generally, of course, it's the latter. But we now know that we can exert a lot of influence on this process, and almost all of us are already doing at least *something* to improve our health.

Everything *is either growing or decaying.*
That includes our health.

Maybe we're trying to eat well. Or we're trying to exercise more often. Or we're attempting to sleep better. Few people do all these things as well as we might, but almost all of us are doing *something*, which means we're doing something that we can build upon.

These are the initiating tailwinds of hyper wellness—the starting places from which we can best build momentum. From there, we can better access our secondary tailwinds—the things that we might not be doing yet to increase our momentum toward hyper wellness, but that becomes more possible once we've already got a little bit of wind in our sails.

There is no one, at any age, or in any state of wellness, who cannot access their tailwinds or benefit from them. But it's also true that it's easier to gain and maintain momentum when you are biologically younger and healthier. The trick is that this is also the time in many of our lives in which we are also more resilient, and thus it feels like we don't need to diet, exercise, sleep, and reduce negative stress—let alone diet *more*, exercise *more*, or sleep *more*. But the earlier we invest in finding and maintaining these wellness-promotive elements of our lives, the easier it will be to ride those winds long into a healthy and happy future.

Eating Habits

Here's the least surprising thing we'll write in this entire book: A good diet is essential to wellness. Everyone knows this, and yet most people find it hard to stick to a healthy way of eating.

All too often, that's because we don't consider a major headwind working against dietary changes: Our bodies are metabolically accustomed to the kinds of fuel we've been using, and substantial changes—even those that may be very healthy in the long term if they can be sustained—throw off that balance, impacting our energy levels, moods, and mental clarity.

That brings us to one of the most important primary principles of identifying and using dietary tailwinds: Don't stage a "diet coup," overthrowing everything about the way you eat all at once. Instead, build upon your initiating tailwinds—those healthy dietary habits you already have.

A lot of people don't think they're doing *anything* right. That's not true. Even people who aren't doing *much* right are usually doing *something* right. By way of example, while few Americans eat as many vegetables as they should, most people do put at least some veggies on their plates, and they know that they would be better off if they ate a few more—and that fusion of doing and knowing is an initiating tailwind.

---

*A lot of people don't think they're doing anything *right*. That's not true.*

We are often suckered into binary, all-or-nothing thinking. For instance, many people recognize that there are a lot of health benefits to vegetarianism, so millions of people try to go cold turkey on meat each year. But guess what? They almost always fail, with lapse rates as high as 84 percent, according to some reports.[13] The shame of this is that there's a whole lot of room between "I'll just keep eating the same pathetic number of veggies I'm eating now" and "I'll never eat meat again."

The vegetables you *already* eat, even in small quantities, are a tailwind—something you're already doing that's good for your health that can be leaned into, just a bit, to get an even bigger advantage. It's hard to completely overhaul a diet, but it's easy to add just one serving of vegetables a day to your usual diet—and that's also a shift that can offer the sort of immediate, palpable, positive feedback so important to the virtuous cycle.

That might seem like a big claim, but researchers from the United Kingdom have demonstrated a striking dose-response association between vegetable consumption and mental well-being,[14] such that just one extra portion of produce a day can offer noticeable, meaningful improvements in mood, which then becomes capacity for other changes.

Of course, increasing vegetables is an almost universally accepted principle of a healthy diet. Other foods can be a lot more complicated. For decades, many physicians recommended that people who are striving for greater fitness should avoid fats at all costs. Then it became conventional wisdom that monounsaturated and polyunsaturated fats are appropriate in moderation, while trans and saturated fats are the things to avoid. And more recently, it's become clear that "moderation" can and should mean different things to different healthy people, and the jury is still out on saturated fats like butter, palm and coconut oils, cheese, and red meat, all of which can be healthy in the right dietary context.[15] As such, it's understandable to not be certain whether your personal fat consumption is a headwind or tailwind—if it's promoting aging or wellness. Similar questions abound for grains (which offer fiber, vitamins, and other nutrients but are often also packed with carbohydrates, which can be valuable in some diets and harmful in others), many fruits (which are also rich in vitamins and often a good source of antioxidants, but can raise blood sugar levels), and potatoes (ditto on vitamins and fiber, but also carbs).

These questions are best answered on an individual basis, which is why *slowly* building toward the principles of a specific diet regimen—rather than switching suddenly as so many failed dieters do—can be an effective way to assess how the elements of that diet impact your wellness. By way of example, if you chose to slowly build toward a Mediterranean diet (one of the most well-studied diets in the world, with copious evidence of its health benefits[16]), you might begin by first adding a daily helping of unprocessed grains, such as barley, bulgur, farro, millet, oats, and spelt. In the long term, these foods have been associated with reductions in coronary heart disease, cardiovascular disease, cancer, and diabetes, but of course you're not going to notice any of that right away. What you are likely to notice, even following a single meal, is the sensation of greater satiation—whole grains are very filling—and thus a reduction in the urge to eat other, less healthy foods.

It can nonetheless be hard to conceptualize how these minute changes are helping you move toward greater healthfulness. Indeed, even when the steps we take are positive, if they are small compared to our lofty ambitions, they can feel like failures. But a friend of ours, Peotr, is a good example of why this isn't the case.

In 2022, Peotr's goal was to lose 25 pounds. He understood that was a lot of weight to drop, but he also reasoned—rationally—that about 2 pounds each month was an achievable goal.

"I lost a little initially, gained some back, lost a little more, and so on," Peotr told us. "By summertime it was clear I wasn't going to hit my goal, but I still tried for the rest of the year."

When that year came to an end, Peotr had lost just 5 pounds.

Is that a failure? No. It's a weaker tailwind, but it's a tailwind nonetheless.

This becomes crystal clear when you think in a physiologically holistic way about what happens with just five pounds of weight loss. With each step Peotr took, he was asking his body to exert 5 pounds less strain on his knees, hips, and spine. And if you want to put into perspective how much a difference this can make over the thousands of steps you take each day, simply put a two-liter bottle of water into a backpack and carry it around from sunrise to sunset. By the end of the day, that little bit of added weight (about 4.4 pounds) will contribute to palpable energy loss and likely even some pain. Five pounds matters!

This is the way we should think about dietary changes and results that bring us toward greater healthfulness. Each positive step, no matter how incremental, counts!

It's important to note that some dietary lifestyles—keto being perhaps the most prominent example—are incumbent on all-or-nothing approaches, thus preclusive of a slow-build strategy. A reduction in just one source of carbohydrates or simple sugars won't result in ketosis, the metabolic state that occurs when fat, rather than glucose, becomes the body's primary source of energy. Keto can be tremendously effective for some people, but it does have a high failure rate, likely in part because it won't work unless someone is all in.

Each positive step, no matter how incremental, counts!

Other diets are also likely to have greater impact on holistic health when enacted in their entirety. For reasons that are not yet completely understood, the whole is greater than the parts of eating approaches like the Mediterranean diet.[17] But almost every element of that diet is beneficial all by itself. Adding more whole grains to your diet is healthy irrespective of just about anything else you do. Replacing red and processed meat with fatty fish like salmon, mackerel, and tuna can make a significant difference in your risk of heart disease, cancer, and other diseases.[18] A daily helping of legumes—beans, peas, and lentils—is not just one of the greatest predictors of long-term health,[19] but also offers immediately palpable benefits, particularly in terms of providing a long boost of energy as a result of slowly digested carbohydrates.

If you're not sure what to add or subtract, or what diet to build toward, there are three basic principles that all "good" diets share:

- Eat whole foods.
- Treat food as fuel.
- Don't overconsume.

What are you doing already in alignment with one or more of these principles? That's a tailwind. Now, accentuate it.

Others might quibble. They might say, "That's not enough." They're wrong. What matters is what is sustainable and buildable. On the virtuous cycle, no step in the right direction is too small.

Exercise

When we exercise, we sleep better. When we exercise, we gain energy. When we exercise, we prevent disease. And when we sleep better, have more energy, and prevent disease, we build capacity to engage in the parts of our lives that bring meaning and joy. Ergo, exercise is among the most powerful of tailwinds.

It's also an initiating tailwind—something almost certainly part of your life already, even if it feels as though you haven't engaged in intentional exercise in years. That's because, just as almost everyone is already doing something positive relative to how they eat that can be built upon for a greater effect, almost everyone is already getting some degree of exercise that can be accentuated for greater gains. We'll dive more deeply into this idea in chapter 10, but it may be good to offer some concrete examples of how this principle works to improve upon existing tailwinds.

Although Americans lag behind many other nations in terms of mobility, the average US adult takes roughly 5,000 steps a day,[20] the equivalent of about two miles of walking. Little of this comes as the result of intentionally exertive exercise, but from a tailwinds perspective that doesn't matter. Owing to the steps they take to move about their homes, get to work, and run their daily errands, most people are at least halfway to the 10,000 daily steps that are often recommended as a good target for basic daily mobility—although 7,000[21] to 7,500[22] seem to be the "sweet spot" beyond which wellness benefits appear to level out, which means a lot of us are more than two-thirds of the way to a very good goal!

There are two easy ways to accentuate this existing tailwind: walking more and walking faster. A team of researchers from Denmark and Australia demonstrated that when a person adds just 2,000 extra steps a day to the activity they're already engaged in, they lower their risk of premature death by more than 8 percent.[23] The same scientists discovered that people who walk at a brisker pace are also less likely to suffer from long-term health problems.[24] These consequential tailwind accentuators can be achieved through simple shifts toward intentionality: parking a little farther away from work each day, taking a quick stroll around the block during a break at work, meeting friends for a "coffee walk" rather than a sit-down visit in a café, and so on.

The same principles apply to whatever deliberately exertive exercise we're already getting. When the National Center for Health Statistics released a major report on how much US adults exercise in 2018, a lot of the focus was on the fact that fewer than a quarter of Americans were getting "enough" of a workout, defined by the Department of Health and Human Services as 150 minutes of moderate physical activity or 75 minutes of vigorous physical activity each week.[25] What was missed in that framing is that the vast majority of people were at least getting *some* deliberate exercise. Long-term polling has shown that most Americans do exercise a few days each week.[26] So, are most of us getting enough exercise? No. But do most of us already have a significant tailwind upon which we can build? Absolutely. And just as "more steps" and "faster steps" are the easiest ways to accentuate the health benefits associated with the passive activity we already get just from going about our lives, "more time" and "more rigor" are the easiest ways to increase the tailwinds when it comes to intentionally exertive exercise, too.

Are most of us getting enough exercise? No. But do most of us already have a significant tailwind upon which we can build? Absolutely.

Remember: Small steps are buildable gains. A 5-minute boost on a 15-minute-per-day jogging habit equates to 30 additional hours of exercise each year. Or, without adding any time at all to a running habit, a pace shift from 4 to 5 miles per hour would add about 90 miles to your total annual mileage. That's greater than the distance you would run if you participated in three marathons!

Some people might say, "But I just don't like running." There are two good answers to that protestation.

The first, and easiest, is to recognize that running, while arguably the simplest and most accessible way to exercise, is far from the only way to exercise. And since there is no better motivator than enjoyment, the appropriate question to ask is: What *do* you like doing? Is it basketball? Fantastic. Is it lifting weights? Great. Is it jumping rope or playing pickleball or boxing? Wonderful. If it increases your heart rate when you do it, and you enjoy it, then accentuating this initiating tailwind is simply a matter of more time and more rigor.

Some people don't like *any* kind of exercise, or the kinds of athletic activities they've most enjoyed in the past—soccer or ultimate Frisbee or windsurfing or whatever—are no longer accessible. When this is the case, exercises like jogging, yoga, and calisthenics are almost always going to be the best step forward regardless of whether one enjoys those exercises. In instances like this, "more time" and "more rigor" requires a mindset shift: There are plenty of things in our lives we don't enjoy doing but we choose to do because they are important. So, if you can't make exercise fun, at least acknowledge its importance and make the choice to do it anyway.

That's not a big ask. Not at first, at least. You don't have to choose to start running a marathon. Or a 5K. Or even a single loop around your block. All you have to do to initiate a tailwind is choose to do a little more than what you're doing right now.

Sleep

When we get better sleep, we have more energy. When we get better sleep, our moods improve. When we get better sleep, we make better decisions. And yet, by and large, our sleep habits are atrocious. And while most people seem to understand that they need more sleep, few seem to grasp that it's just as important (and a lot of emerging research suggests it's far more important) to improve the *quality* of their sleep. This is a subject we will discuss in chapter 7. But since sleep is one of the things that we all do, it's also an important example of a primary tailwind—and an aspect of wellness that many people don't understand very well.

Sleep quantity—that good old eight-hours-a-night standard—is just one element of sleep quality, which can be evaluated in terms of the depth of sleep and types of brain activities, and the resultant effects on alertness, intellect, and emotion. Indeed, eight hours in bed is meaningless if it's not followed by clarity, insight, and contentment. And yet, until recently, most studies and doctors' recommendations have centered on the number of hours people sleep, and few other factors.[27]

The truth is that it's not about the *number* of hours nearly so much as it is about the hours at which each night of sleep begins and ends—because our evolutionary programming was set by millions of years of sleep and wake patterns aligned to 24-hour cycles including some daylight and some darkness. During the vast majority of that time, circadian predictability was the rule. Thus, if you average just 5 hours of sleep each 24-hour cycle, but those hours sometimes come early, sometimes come late, and are sometimes broken into pieces, you can improve upon the quality, and thus healthfulness, of your sleep without adding a single minute to your slumber, so long as you start and end close to the same times every day.

Getting on a steady cycle is a matter of adhering to both a set bedtime and fixed wake-up time, but of the two of these variables, the second is far more important. That's because—thanks to time-settable alarms—we have a lot more control over the moment we get up than the moment we fall asleep, no matter what time we *try* to go to sleep.

As is the case with diets and exercise, the odds of success via a "sleep coup" are low. Strengthening this tailwind is a matter of making gradual adjustments, perceiving the benefits, and investing that capacity into more adjustments. That's important when it comes to establishing bedtimes and waking times, but also for the other elements of "sleep hygiene," the behavioral and environmental practices surrounding our sleep, like cool room temperatures, clean and comfortable bedding, buffers for outside noises, and the elimination of artificial light, the latter of which is perhaps the most widely violated principle, particularly because we're surrounded by backlit screens from smartphones, computers, and televisions. Indeed, surveys have shown most Americans are staring at one of these sources of artificial light within an hour of going to bed, and many people look at screens when they're actively trying to sleep! The result is a suppression of the production of melatonin, which is evolutionarily designed to trigger tiredness when the sun sets, and a resultant incapacity to get to sleep as fast as we should and to sleep as deeply as we should.[28]

The ultimate goal should be to keep backlit screens out of the bedroom and away from our eyes at least an hour before we go to bed. But let's assess the realism of that goal: If we offered you an extra month's wages if, starting today, you banned screens from your bedroom and never watched TV, worked on the computer, or looked at your phone an hour before your bedtime every night, for a year, would you succeed? You probably wouldn't, and neither would we! And honestly, we don't know anyone who would. So even though those practices would improve nearly everyone's health, it's a moot point.

But when it comes to sleep, minutes matter. And gradual movements toward a goal like that can pay huge dividends.

That's what Parker learned.

"I don't think there has been a single night of my life since I was a teenager that I didn't fall asleep with the television on," he said. "When I was young, I'd just throw on HBO and fall asleep to whatever movie was playing, which was usually a movie I'd seen ten times before, so it was sort of soothing. Then Netflix came along and I'd just turn on the same show every night. I've probably watched every episode of *The Office* 400 times. I don't even laugh at the jokes anymore. I know them all. And that's what makes it so good as a sleep aid."

Parker knew it was bad for him, but there was no way he was going to break that habit all at once, or ever. "People might say, 'But how do you know if you don't try?' and that's fair, I guess, but I can't even imagine trying," he said.

Parker had been on the virtuous cycle for about a year—realizing gradual gains in health and energy related mainly to food and exercise—when it occurred to him he could apply some of the capacity he'd earned toward the goal of reducing his nighttime light exposure. "I was only watching Netflix anyway," he said. "So I didn't need to have that on the TV in my room. I put it on my laptop, which is obviously a smaller screen, so that logically meant less light."

After a few days, he removed the TV altogether. And a few weeks later he made another change—instead of playing *The Office* on his computer, he played it on his phone. "So, that was even less light," he said. "And maybe it's just in my head, but it does feel like it was making a difference in how fast I was getting to sleep and how rested I was the next day."

Shortly after moving his nighttime watching to his phone, Parker learned he could set a timer to turn off the show after he fell asleep. And eventually he learned he didn't need the screen on at all—it was the voices that were helping lull him to sleep each night.

In 2021, Netflix dropped *The Office* from its streaming service. "When that happened, I briefly considered that it might be time to finally break the habit," he said. "But instead I just dropped Netflix and bought the whole series so I don't have to pay for a streaming service for a single show that I only listen to for, like, seven minutes before I fall asleep each night."

That's the imperfect but *much better* place he was at the last time we checked in with him.

"There's still no way I'm going to turn it off altogether—and, yeah, I understand that having extra noise is bad for sleep quality, too. I'm not in denial about any of this," he said. "But I also don't have any doubt that I'm a hundred times better off right now than before. I know that eliminating that source of light, which used to be on all night long, is better for me, and I can tangibly feel the difference in my life."

Those *tangible* differences are what we're trying to accentuate—no matter which tailwind we are trying to capture. There is no question that reducing light sources before sleep improves sleep quality at a neurological level, but if those improvements aren't at least faintly perceptible at a conscious level, too, you'll have a much harder time putting those gains to use in the form of further positive actions.

Those tangible *differences are what we're trying to accentuate.*

And as it turns out, one of the most tangible tailwinds is something that, for many people, first seems to be a substantial headwind.

Time... Again

It took a global pandemic for Caishen, a Restore client from Chicago, where he works in manufacturing sales, to discover that time was a hugely untapped tailwind.

"Not having enough time is a huge excuse," Caishen said. "That might be hard for a lot of people to hear. It was hard for me to accept. Really, two years ago, if you'd told me that, I would have wanted to punch you because my life felt so busy. And that's why I didn't make time for the things that I knew I needed to do to be healthy."

For the first five years of his career, Caishen was constantly on the road. "I was eating in restaurants almost every night because I felt like I didn't have time. I wasn't exercising because I felt like I didn't have time. I was only getting four or five hours of sleep at night because I felt like I didn't have time."

Then the COVID-19 pandemic hit, and Caishen's travels stopped for more than a year.

"All of a sudden, I had all this time," he said. "But guess what? I didn't get healthy. I ordered take-out food and I still didn't exercise and I was still sleeping poorly. And that's when it occurred to me: It wasn't time. It was me. I wasn't using my time wisely."

He wasn't alone. Nearly half of Americans gained unhealthy weight during the first year of the pandemic.[29] Despite the fact that many people had more time owing to eliminated commutes and canceled social events, they were actually getting less exercise overall.[30] Many people who were working from home weren't walking as much. Those who had been going to the gym didn't replace that habit with other forms of exercise. And long-COVID symptoms prevented some people from getting back into their prepandemic exercise habits.

There are lots of people who are legitimately strapped for time. But for most people, a lack of spare time isn't actually a headwind at all. Most people have plenty of time that could be used to accentuate other tailwinds; they just don't use it for that purpose. Indeed, researchers who track and study the way people utilize spare time—an average of five hours of it per day, according to an analysis of the American Time Use Survey—found that instead of using our time to shop for healthier foods, cook healthier meals, take more steps, engage in more exertive exercise, or get better sleep, we hand over the majority of that time to our various screens, engaging in excessive game-playing, show-watching, and social media–scrolling. "There is a general perception among the public and even public health professionals that a lack of leisure time is a major reason that Americans do not get enough physical activity," Deborah Cohen, a coauthor of the study, said in 2019. "But we found no evidence for those beliefs."[31]

When he came face-to-face with the realization that it wasn't just his busy schedule that was preventing him from being healthier, Caishen evaluated the ways he was using his time, keeping a log of the shows he was watching and using an app that tracked the time he was spending online. "I was spending almost three hours every day online watching, reading, and chatting with other people about sports on social media, and on the weekends it was even more than that," he said. "I did the math. That was like six or seven weeks of my life, every year."

Caishen still loves sports, especially college football and basketball. But he now schedules his viewing and chatting. "I keep it to two hours each day," he says. "If I want to watch a game that's going to be longer than that, I cut back another day to make it happen. That's still a ton of time, but it's a lot less than what I was doing, and I think I'm ready to cut back a little more."

The hour each day he has gained has been reinvested into exercise. And even though he's been back on the road for several years—and is now traveling even more than he did before—he no longer feels like he's strapped for time. "I hit the gym first thing when I get checked into the hotel, and I always choose hotels that are either close to a grocery store where I can get fresh food or close to a restaurant that has healthy options," he said. "And instead of turning on *SportsCenter* at the end of the day, I check in on one of the college sports message boards that I'm still active on, then turn off my computer and read a few pages of a book before I go to sleep. The TV stays off."

Many people are like Caishen: Time isn't really the problem. The way we *use* time is. But when we replace unhealthy activities with fundamentally healthy ones like exercise, healthy eating, and better sleep, the result is *more* energy. That means a greater capacity to focus, which means improved effectiveness and efficiency at the things that we actually have to do, which in turn means more time to do the things we want to do! The reallocation of spare time from "time sinks" to "energy accentuators" is a gift that keeps on giving—a tailwind that most people don't even realize they have.

Time isn't really the problem. The way we use time is.

It's Elemental

Once we have taken a census of our health, and understand the headwinds and tailwinds that are most influential in our lives, we can explore ways to impact the directionality and momentum of aging and wellness.

There are endless ways to think about this process, but we've found the most effective framework is through the nine elements of hyper wellness: cold, heat, oxygen, hydration, rest, light, nourishment, movement, and connection. Each of the therapies we will discuss in this book is aligned to one or more of these elements, and designed to result in an immediately visceral impact that will push you further toward the goal of hyper wellness.

Positive engagement of any one of the nine elements, by itself, should get you moving in the right direction. Many of the elements can be coupled to provide an even more profound impact. Some of the elements (cold and heat, in particular) can be contrasted for a greater effect. There is no "right order" or "correct combination," so we encourage you to explore the next nine chapters as you see fit, commensurate with your interest in each of these component parts of holistic wellness.

We implore you, however, to make it your ultimate goal to incorporate all of these elements into your life in a meaningful way. Those who do are virtually locked into the virtuous cycle of feeling better and doing more, which is the path to hyper wellness.

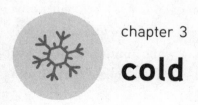

chapter 3

cold

For more than 10 years, Rachelle had been living with the knowledge that she had multiple sclerosis, and she understood what that meant for her future.

There is no cure for MS. Not yet, anyway. And so Rachelle knew that, over time, she was likely to experience increasingly frequent pain, tremors, and difficulties controlling her muscles, among other symptoms of an immune disorder that progressively attacks the layers of protein and fat that sheath the nerves of the brain and spinal cord.

But even though she knew about all the devastating possibilities, the morning she awoke unable to move came as a blow.

"I woke up after riding my bike 40 miles that weekend," she said. "I couldn't feel from the waist down. And I mean, like, I couldn't feel anything."

Overnight, her life had changed. While she would regain feeling in her legs following that acute period of paralysis, the debilitating symptoms of MS were no longer a frightening, foreboding possibility, but a reality. Bike riding became difficult, and on some days unthinkable. It was no longer a certainty that she would begin each day by taking her two golden retrievers on a walk around her neighborhood in Austin. Just putting on her clothes could now be a painful ordeal. Travel, which was a big part of her job, seemed like it would forever be prohibitively hard.

At that time, Rachelle's goal was to continue doing the things she loved—as much as she could and for as long as possible—before her mobility became even more limited. That would necessitate finding a way to keep involuntary muscle contractions at bay, while limiting her pain and preserving her energy enough so that she could continue to stretch and exercise.

For Rachelle, cryotherapy was the key—and, despite her initial trepidation, she soon became a devotee.

Almost everyone feels a little bit nervous before their first experience with whole-body cryo, and that's a reasonable emotional response. After all, there is nothing in our natural world that comes anywhere close to the negative 150 degrees Fahrenheit and colder temperatures that occur in a cryo chamber. (The known natural record, set in 2007 in Vostok, Antarctica, was negative 128.6 degrees Fahrenheit.) But the rewards for getting over that initial trepidation are vast, because of what happens inside our bodies when we get really cold.

It all starts in the skin—where, in just a few minutes, temperatures can drop 50 to 60 degrees Fahrenheit, activating a fight-or-flight response in the roughly 35 billion cells that make up the largest organ in our bodies. These cells—programmed to be sentries against all sorts of external stresses—release a combination of signaling proteins into the blood that is moving through every inch of our skin at all times. These signals quickly reach the brain, which responds by releasing chemical messengers like norepinephrine, which transmits even more vigilance-directing signals to nerve, muscle, and gland cells throughout the rest of the body. With that, every system of the body is placed on high alert.

This is not unlike what happens in a joint military exercise, where multiple service branches—and hundreds of divisions under each of those branches—work together to ensure they are adequately communicating, using effective tactics, and ready for surprises, but without having to engage in actual combat operations. Likewise, cryotherapy is an opportunity for all the different tissues and systems in our bodies to coordinate against a perceived threat, albeit a threat that is temporary and, experienced in moderation, very safe.

Cryotherapy is an opportunity for all the different tissues and systems in our bodies to coordinate against a perceived threat.

For Rachelle, cryo has been so successful that her goal is no longer simply staying out of a wheelchair. Today, she is living life to its fullest, just as she was before that terrifying morning when she woke up unable to move.

Now, on the day after a cryo session, "I wake up and I feel so much better, with so much less pain," she said. "I can continue to do the things I want to."

Maximizing Mobility

The therapy that eventually changed Rachelle's life, and so many others', came about in no small part because of the work of a pioneering physical therapist named Maggie Knott and a relentless neurologist named Sedgwick Mead. In the 1960s, Knott and Mead had begun exploring the use of topical cryotherapy for patients suffering from spasticity disorders, including MS, at the Kaiser Foundation Rehabilitation Center in Vallejo, California. Back then, the most common method of physical therapy preparation for those who were about to undergo assisted stretching and exercise was heating in a warm whirlpool bath. The idea behind this practice was that the heat would prepare a person's muscles and joints, but

Knott and Mead were frustrated because it didn't work all that well. They correctly recognized that these baths did not result in a significant shift in heat exchange—not even at skin level—so the deep tissue effects were minimal.

But what if they took their patients in the opposite direction? By soaking towels in ice water and then wrapping the towels around the part of the body that was being targeted for stretching, Knott and Mead discovered they could dramatically shift the temperature of targeted tissues. That might not loosen the muscles and joints for stretching and exercise, as warm water was at least intended to do, but perhaps it would create an anesthetic effect, giving patients greater capacity to work through the pain of physical therapy.

And it worked—if only for a short time.

"Resistance to passive stretch may melt away under the effects of ice packs," they later wrote, "but this effect is gone in a few hours or a day."

Those precious hours, though, provided a vital window of opportunity for intervention. Their patients were able to do more stretching and exercising, keeping joints more nimble, preventing muscle atrophy, and providing a boost of strength and endurance. Patients "who may lie comatose for days or weeks in flexion postures," Knott and Mead observed, "may be preserved from irreversible contracture by brief ice packing and a little stretching just once a day."[1]

It was a right-away intervention with life-changing results!

While they figured that their method of icing was having an anesthetic effect on superficial nerves, Knott and Mead also suspected there must be another mechanistic mystery at play. At the time, however, they didn't have any leads as to what it might be. But after seeing the power of this process on their patients for many years, they understood that the effect was more important than the cause. In 1966, they published an account of their work in a small, regional medical journal, and while the publication was relatively obscure, the report gained the attention of physicians and physical therapists around the globe who were desperate to identify ways to help their patients resist the ravages of MS. Ice-packing became a common part of care.

During most of the 1970s, '80s, and '90s, however, there was little further research into the use of topical cold therapy for MS patients. Clinicians knew it worked, but they didn't know why, and there was little exploration of ways to take this form of therapy to the next level.

Something shifted in the early 2000s, though, as a generation of researchers trained at the School of Cryotherapy at the Academy of Physical Education in Wrocław, Poland, began to spread out around the globe, taking with them their ever-deepening expertise in the clinical impacts of whole-body cryotherapy, in which a person stands upright in a chamber cooled using liquid nitrogen to temperatures far beyond what could be achieved through ice packing. It would be a vast overstatement to suggest that research on cryotherapy for MS patients became commonplace, but after a period of time in which the connection was noted a few times per decade in obscure academic publications, now multiple articles were being released each year, in increasingly prestigious medical journals. Researchers were building upon the early observations of clinicians like Knott and Mead and were beginning to offer some explanations for the effects they had long witnessed. Importantly, the research increasingly suggested that it was not just an anesthetic effect that was permitting greater flexibility and improved exercise. For instance, by analyzing recordings of the electrical activity produced in the muscle tissue of MS patients who had undergone cryotherapy, researchers discovered a striking increase in muscle extension and an equally striking decrease in muscle contraction; the bioelectrical muscle activity itself had been impacted by the cryo, leading to less muscular fatigue[2] and thus greater capacity to engage in more exercise. Patients felt better, so they could do more. They did more, and so they felt better.

This brings us back to Rachelle. She has resumed traveling for work—so long as she knows she can access cryo while she is on the road. "My first question," she said, "is always 'Do we have a Restore there?' Because I need to go there."

That's music to our ears, and not simply because it demonstrates a customer's positive experiences with our company. That part is nice, of course, but Rachelle's desire—and indeed, her need—to be close to a Restore studio speaks to the importance of reaching more people! And yes, that's a business-oriented goal—it would be disingenuous not to acknowledge that—but we've also come to see it as a social responsibility. Multiple sclerosis affects approximately 400,000 people in the United States and a proportional population of many millions of people around the globe. Research suggests that almost all these individuals could benefit from access to cryotherapy,[3] not just as a temporary mitigative measure for pain and mobility, but as an essential starting point in the feel-better-do-more cycle leading to hyper wellness.

If we discovered that cryo was effective only for those with MS and no one else, the chance to help people like Rachelle would be enough for us to continue onward toward the goal of ensuring that safe, affordable, accessible cryotherapy services were available everywhere. But that's not where this story ends.

A Focus on Athletic Recovery

Long before we had a name for our company, long before we'd hired a single employee, and long before we even considered where our first center would be located, we had a pretty good idea of who our core customer would be. And while we knew that cryotherapy had applications for people with autoimmune diseases, understood that it would draw some thrill-seekers, and recognized that it was falsely but increasingly being viewed as a cure-all by affluent alternative-health adherents, we felt strongly that—if we could improve upon the retail cryotherapy experience—the average customer would be a middle-aged athlete seeking to accelerate the process of recovery. That, we believed, would be our "bread and butter."

Our surety was both market-based and science-based. Cold immersion has long been used by elite athletes to reduce muscle pain and soreness after training and competition. And cold therapy is becoming more common even for nonprofessional athletes; these days, many high schoolers are familiar with the constant electrical humming and periodic crashing noises emanating from the industrial ice machine in their locker rooms—right next to the stainless-steel tub where football, soccer, and basketball players line up to take a frigid plunge after competitions. Somewhat fancier versions of these tanks can be found in nearly every professional sports training room, and it's not uncommon for athletes to take post-game questions from sports journalists while sitting in an ice tub—anesthetizing acute pain, stimulating cellular activity to help in the repair of the tears that occur in muscle fibers during intense exercise, and constricting blood vessels to flush out waste products such as lactic acid that build during lengthy periods of competition.[4]

Amateur athletes have always looked to professionals for guidance. Indeed, there is a global market based on this fundamental fact. Few of us can hit a golf ball like Rory McIlroy, but we can use the same TaylorMade driver in his bag. Most folks can't fight like mixed martial artist Amanda Nunes, but we can wear the same style of Reeboks she trains in. Not many recreational soccer players can bend it like Catarina Macario, but they can lace up the same Adidas cleats she wears. And this is true when it comes to recovery, too. As Tom Brady moved across the public consciousness from being a very good quarterback to being a very good and very old quarterback, Under Armour recognized a unique branding opportunity. Most of us wouldn't get up easily—or at all—after being knocked down by an NFL defensive lineman, let alone more than 500 times, as Brady has over the course of his long career, but for about $200 we can sleep in the same specially designed "recovery pajamas" that Brady reportedly wears each night.

There have been attempts to make an ice-cold bath as common as a daily shower. One of the most entertaining segments in the history of the popular business reality series *Shark Tank* came in the spring of 2022 when co-host and angel investor Robert Herjavec shrieked his way though a few frigid minutes in a Plunge brand bath. That may be an option for a small segment of the population, but at a starting price of $5,000, it's not for most people. And while "cold bath houses" are relatively common along the ocean coastlines and on the edges of inland lakes in Sweden, there doesn't appear to be a viable way to duplicate that sort of ocean-dipping experience in most places in the United States. So, in most cases, ice baths aren't one of the things that amateur athletes can do "just like the pros." And even those who do have the ability to ice bathe without too much trouble often find the experience to be unpleasant, even once they've been doing it for a long time. It's something they dread, not something they look forward to.

Among the people in the room during that hilarious *Shark Tank* segment, however, was Mark Cuban, the owner of the National Basketball Association's Dallas Mavericks—one of the first professional teams to adopt whole-body cryotherapy. The Mavs' director of player health and performance, Casey Smith, was able to convince then–point guard Jason Kidd to try it for the first time in 2011. Kidd was immediately sold on the experience, and helped convert Jason Terry, Dirk Nowitzki, Shawn Marion, and others to the practice.

That year the Mavericks won the NBA championship.

"We thought it was our secret weapon," Kidd said, "because of what it did and how it made everyone feel."[5]

While Kidd correctly predicted that cryo chambers would soon be "in every locker room and probably on every campus because of what it does to the body and how you feel and the success rate it's had so far," that sort of endorsement wouldn't have meant much to the general public if cryo was economically or functionally prohibitive. But at the same time as a wave of enthusiasm for cryo was washing over the NBA and other professional sports leagues, mavericks of a different sort were flooding the zone with relatively cheap cryotherapy machines that could be installed almost anywhere.

Indeed, at that time, if you had a few thousand dollars, a reliable source for liquid nitrogen, and a space the size of a closet, you could be in the cryotherapy business in a matter of days. Soon, fly-by-night cryo centers were popping up everywhere. In one Southern California beach town, for instance, a local boot merchant converted a dressing room into a cryo chamber, and there may never be a better symbol for the sorts of anarchic business environments that come about when a new technology meets public enthusiasm. It truly was the wild west.

None of this would have meant anything to us, though, if whole-body cryotherapy didn't actually work to help athletes recover. After all, there have been plenty of health and wellness trends that started in professional locker rooms that were simply bunk. Back in the early 2000s, for instance, lots of pro athletes—especially baseball players, it seemed—began wearing colorful vinyl necklaces embedded with titanium that some believed would "produce an electrical charge that relieves pain, increases energy, and speeds recovery."[6] At one time hundreds of Major League Baseball players were wearing these things. Not so much these days.

Hype is not a business plan. Good science can be, though. And to that end, the research backing clinically administered whole-body cryotherapy for athletic recovery is compelling. In one randomized control trial of experienced runners published in 2011, those who received whole-body cryotherapy recovered far faster than those who were treated in other ways.[7] A year later, a separate research group published a study showing that tennis players who received cryo treatments twice a day over five consecutive days during a training camp had a 60 percent decrease in proinflammatory protein signalers and a 30 percent increase in anti-inflammatory protein signalers in their bloodstream than those who didn't receive the same treatment.[8] Another year down the road, a third independent group of researchers published a study showing that cryo administered before exercise helped a group of male professional volleyball players maintain lower levels of inflammation.[9] And one more year past that, researchers found that whole-body cryo was an effective way to reduce both inflammation and cholesterol levels following intensive exercise.[10] So, by the time we began investigating cryotherapy in 2015, we were confident that it wasn't just a passing athletic fad. The research that has been conducted since that time on the impacts has only bolstered this confidence.[11]

Hype is not a business plan. Good science can be, though.

The key is translating this science to the real world—so the operative question is "Are our clients seeing the same results as subjects in these studies?" And when it comes to athletic recovery, the answer is "Absolutely."

Shawn, a former professional football player, is an excellent example. After a career that included starting positions on multiple teams in the NFL, Shawn moved to Austin to be close to many good friends and family members. And although he was no longer training in the same ways he had when preparing to play before tens of thousands of people each Sunday of the season, his daily workout regimen remained intense by pretty much anyone else's standards.

"I had been introduced to cold therapy in my college days, and it was a big part of my recovery regimen for my whole career," he told us in the fall of 2022. "What I didn't expect was that I'd still need it after downshifting, but I still get sore and I'm still carrying a lot of the damage that was done to my body over the years, so I found my way back to ice baths and the cryo spa. I'm a pretty big believer in what it does for me both physically to reduce inflammation and mentally to keep me motivated the next day to go at it again in the gym."

So, it turns out we were partially right. Many of our customers have turned out to be athletes. Professionals, Olympians, and amateurs. High schoolers developing their skills and senior citizens who have been playing their sport for decades. And there are plenty of people who are just like we were when we started this journey—middle-aged athletes who wanted to keep running, biking, swimming, or pursuing some other athletic passion. These are exactly the folks we figured Restore would be serving when we opened our first studio. But, as you already know, that's also not where things ended.

Fighting Chronic Pain

Among the most frequent users of cryotherapy, and those for whom the research of efficacy is most robust, are individuals suffering from fibromyalgia, also known as chronic pain syndrome. About 3 percent of people have fibromyalgia, with women disproportionately affected, and there is no cure.

There's also no consensus on why fibromyalgia occurs. Some recent studies, however, have homed in on the activity of cytokines—small proteins that travel in the bloodstream, mediating cellular communication, and playing a key role in triggering inflammation.[12] Armed with previous studies that showed that cytokines are often dysregulated in people with fibromyalgia, researchers in Germany sought to understand what would happen to these cellular signalers under cryotherapy, so they invited 23 fibromyalgia patients and 30 healthy control subjects to undergo six weekly sessions of whole-body cryo. The patients reported notable reductions in pain—an effect that became most pronounced after three sessions and that continued for up to three months after the therapy was discontinued. And when the fibromyalgia patients' blood work was analyzed, it turned out that they also had significantly different levels of, and changes to, their cytokines.[13]

A lot of additional study will be needed to understand whether cytokines are the primary culprits in fibromyalgia. What we can say right now—without any doubt and without the need for any further research—is that many people who have spent years suffering from fibromyalgia are finding relief in cryo that they haven't been able to find elsewhere.

"Talking to doctors, every suggestion was medication," said Jackie, who was first diagnosed with fibromyalgia when she was just 17 years old.

But Jackie didn't want to simply manage her pain. After 20 years of that approach, she understood the toll that drugs can take over time. "That was not a road I wanted to go back down," she said. "So, I needed to find something that could help heal my body and make me feel better."

She did. Jackie's regimen includes regular whole-body cryotherapy sessions, followed by a localized cryo, in which a technician directs a hyper-cooled forced-air stream onto targeted areas of the body—a less-studied[14] form of cryo that appears to be especially helpful for those who have specific areas of acute pain.

The results that Jackie has experienced are not unusual, and not limited to a reduction in pain. After cryotherapy, many people with fibromyalgia report having less fatigue, fewer sleep problems, reduced anxiety, better-managed depression, less difficulty concentrating, and improved memory. Is cryo having a direct impact on all those conditions? Probably not. But dealing with chronic pain from day to day is a little like carrying a bag that unexpectedly varies in weight from heavy to very heavy, and from very heavy to unbearable. If you had to shoulder such a burden, every minute of every day, what impact would that have on other areas of your physical and mental health?

Imagine how your body would feel if you were finally able to put that bag down. Imagine what you could do. Imagine the relief you'd experience. That's how it feels to have chronic pain alleviated, even if the effect is temporary. That's the power of the feel-better-do-more cycle.

Skin Health

It has been a few years since the name Bryson Doyle first came to our attention. We'll never forget it.

Most kids who suffer from eczema, a type of atopic dermatitis, try to hide it, but Bryson isn't most kids. The Michigan native was about nine years old when he began a social media campaign to share tips for living with severe food allergies and severe eczema, publicly using his own journey to help destigmatize these conditions for other children.

Part of that journey included cryotherapy. In most circumstances, children are prohibited from whole-body cryo, but when Bryson turned 12, he received permission from his medical care team to use cryo to treat the dry, itchy, and inflamed skin that would often keep him up through the night, especially during Detroit's infamously muggy summers. After Bryson's first session, "he was able to sleep through the night for the first time in months," his mother, Lynell, explained in 2021. "It made him comfortable, reduced his pain, and reduced his need to itch his skin, and all of that helped his skin heal."[15]

A better night of sleep might seem like a relatively minor outcome, but it's important to consider what that means as the starting place for holistic wellness. Black children like Bryson are more likely to suffer from eczema and may also be more likely to suffer from severe flare-ups than white children, but researchers at the University of Pennsylvania have found that Black kids are 30 percent less likely to see a doctor for the condition.[16] That means they're less likely to get the relief they need, which is one of the many reasons that they are more likely to miss school, sometimes to the point of chronic absenteeism.[17] So what we're talking about here isn't just some temporary pain relief—although that alone should be enough. Rather, it's the start of a cycle that starts with right-away wellness, building capacity for other, vitally important opportunities.

A better night of sleep might seem like a relatively minor outcome, but it's important to consider what that means as the starting place for holistic wellness.

Is that a well-stretched extrapolation? If we were only talking about Bryson, then absolutely. We've learned enough about this young man to feel very confident that he's going to have an amazingly successful life. But atopic dermatitis affects up to 20 percent of children.[18] That's tens of millions of kids in the United States and hundreds of millions around the world. So, at a population health level, it's not at all hyperbole to say that increased access to cryotherapy for children suffering from atopic dermatitis could result in countless lives that are changed for the better.

Physicians are increasingly advising their patients to try cryo to treat skin conditions—and even writing prescriptions for younger patients who might not otherwise be permitted to use it. That's especially the case when all pharmaceutical avenues have been exhausted—or when the remaining roads are prohibitively expensive.

Take, for instance, the monoclonal antibody known as Dupixent, jointly developed by Regeneron Pharmaceuticals and Sanofi at a cost of more than $100 million. For people who have exhausted every other drug for severe eczema without finding relief, Dupixent is priceless. The only problem is, of course, that it's not priceless—when the drug debuted following FDA approval in 2017, its listed price was $37,000 a year. Few patients will ever pay that sort of sum out of pocket, of course, but even those who are fortunate enough to have an insurance plan that actually covers Dupixent must cover their deductible, the average family cost of which in 2020 was nearly $8,500 per year.[19]

What's more, no drug, not even one as expensive as Dupixent, is effective on everyone; in its preapproval trials, for instance, Dupixent met the "primary outcome" of helping patients achieve clear or almost clear skin a little more than one third of the time.[20] And no drug is without side effects, either; Dupixent's side effects include pink eye, eyelid inflammation, cornea inflammation, and cold sores on the lips and mouth.

No drug is effective on everyone.
And no drug is without side effects, either.

Likewise, we can't promise that cryotherapy is going to be effective for everyone with every kind of skin condition, or that there are no possible adverse effects. But just as we've seen for cryotherapy's impact on immune diseases and athletic recovery, the research on cryo's effect on dermatitis appears well aligned to the anecdotes. A small clinical study of eczema patients in Finland demonstrated improvements in the extrinsic appearance of the participants' skin, measured skin moisture, hours of sleep, and patient-reported quality of life for those who underwent whole-body cryotherapy three times a week for four weeks.[21] In Korea, a split-body clinical trial, where one side of each patient was treated with localized cryotherapy while the other side was observed as a control, resulted in improvements to skin appearance and reductions in itching.[22] And in Poland, 15 treatments of whole-body cryotherapy resulted in a decrease in eczema intensity and an increase in skin hydration.[23]

It's worth noting that one challenge with cryo studies is that it's hard to create a meaningful placebo-control group. It's hard to fake putting someone through a cryo experience, after all—you know when you're so cold that you're furiously shivering. Without placebo control, it can be a challenge to parcel out the physiological from the psychological. Thus, it's hypothetically possible that the strong effects these studies have demonstrated and the profound improvements cryo users have reported in their own lives could in part be a result of nothing more than each individual's *belief* that the treatment is working.

This would be of less consequence if there was a strong, physiologically mechanistic explanation for why cryo works for dermatitis, but the kinds of studies that would be needed to develop those kinds of conclusions have not been done yet. Thus, we are left with some good assumptions, the strongest of which is that in suppressing inflammation—as cryo has been shown to do in athletic recovery and for patients with multiple sclerosis—extreme cold exposure removes one of the key elements of eczema, which occurs as a result of a combination of genetics, environmental triggers, stress, and immune reaction. And just as fire cannot occur without heat, fuel, and an oxidizing agent, the buffering of inflammation, which is part of the immune reaction, appears to be key to keeping eczema flare-ups at bay.

Could there be a placebo effect at play also? Absolutely. Does that matter? In our minds, not really. When a treatment works, it's appropriate to ask why it works. It's not in anyone's best interest, however, to dismiss or deride something that has been demonstrated to be effective simply because we don't know *why* it's effective.

Over the years, we've met people who are confident that whole-body cryotherapy has been instrumental in their fights against cancer, heart disease, obesity, and even hair loss. The scientific jury is out on all these experiences, and the research may ultimately prove inconclusive. No cryotherapy provider should ever make a health claim that hasn't been backed by science, but we're also not about to argue that these individuals are wrong about the impact cryo has had in their own personal health journeys. Hyper wellness is largely quantitative, but it's also qualitative: How you feel matters. Indeed, it matters more than anything else.

Hyper wellness is largely quantitative, but it's also qualitative: How you feel matters.

Mental and Cognitive Health

Although Poland had long been an epicenter for research on cryotherapy's effect on physical health, this therapy's effects on mental health were often only passingly described in the scientific literature. Doctors in Poland certainly noticed that patients using cryotherapy for mobility, athletic recovery, or pain relief would walk out of a cryo chamber feeling happy, relaxed, refreshed, and even euphoric—but researchers seemed to believe these were little more than side effects of the experience. If your pain has subsided, after all, why *wouldn't* you feel more happy?

Joanna Rymaszewska suspected there was something more at play. Indeed, she argued, there had to be. At the Medical University of Wrocław, where she was a clinical psychiatrist, her patients' improved mental states after cryotherapy often lasted longer than the other improvements that they were experiencing. In 2003, she and her collaborators recruited 23 patients who were regulars at the hospital's depression clinics but had no other medical conditions that would have been previously treated with whole-body cryo. Over two weeks, the patients underwent 10 cryo sessions. Even though she had long suspected there would be a positive effect on the patients' mental health states, Rymaszewska was surprised by the wide-ranging and profound impact the treatments had. In a study such as this, a small effect in most patients, or a large impact on even a few, would have been noteworthy. But Rymaszewska and her colleagues wrote that there had been a beneficial effect to "every patient" in the study.[24] And while each person was affected differently, the net effect was striking. Thoughts of suicide abated. Work life improved. Agitation and anxiety decreased. Interest in sex increased. Worries were diminished.

This was a short-term study with no control arm, but in the two decades that followed, scores of other studies have further supported its key findings with increasingly exacting focuses. In 2019, for instance, Rymaszewska and her collaborators investigated whether whole-body cryotherapy, combined with physical exercise, might help improve the psychological well-being of patients with multiple sclerosis more than exercise alone. It did.[25] In 2020, they looked into cryotherapy as a supplementary therapy for people who were already on drugs to treat their depression. That worked, too.[26] In 2021, they explored whether whole-body cryotherapy, coupled with a computer-based "brain training" regimen, could be a way to help improve the functioning of older adults suffering from cognitive decline. It was.[27]

While Rymaszewska remains a leader in this field, she is no longer a lone pioneer. Research from around the world has affirmed her findings.[28] Yet we're still a long way away from knowing who cryo works best for, under what conditions, and to what extent. As such, the best way to understand the impact of cryotherapy on your own mental health is going to be stepping into a cryo chamber. And unlike pharmaceuticals, which can take a long time to show an impact on a person's mental health, most people will have a sense of whether and how cryo is working for them right away.

That was Anna David's experience. The novelist and podcaster, who has suffered from bouts of depression since her early 20s, first tried cryotherapy when she was in her late 40s. "From the beginning, I felt the immediate euphoria," she later wrote. "I remember chatting with the woman at the front desk after my first treatment and she told me I was grinning ecstatically."[29]

During the first few months of weekly cryotherapy sessions, David suffered a relationship breakup and the death of her cat. It was also winter—a time in which David said she often feels more depressive symptoms. And yet her mood seemed more stable, even buoyant. "The bumps in the road," she explained, "have actually felt just like bumps in the road and not the catastrophic earthquakes similar events have felt like at other times in my life."

It's often said that without mental health, physical health doesn't matter. That's true, but there's more. As anyone who has ever fought against the depressive urge to stay in bed all day can attest, mental health challenges sap us of the resolve to do anything physical—much less the exercise we need to stay fit for life.

Without mental health, physical health is all but impossible. And that's what makes the cryotherapeutic benefits to mental health such a powerful starting place for getting onto the virtuous cycle that leads to hyper wellness. For even if the mental health effects were only short-term, that transitory period of psychological capacity can be parlayed into a series of other beneficial actions with outcomes that can ultimately be felt across an entire lifespan.

Without mental health, physical health is all but impossible.

Freezing Out Aging

It's possible that cryotherapy works *independently* on nervous disorders, athletic recovery, skin conditions, brain function, and other conditions that appear to benefit from this form of treatment. In this way of thinking, the sudden and acute stress response triggered by extreme cold exposure stimulates a different biochemical reaction in different systems.

It's more likely, however, that all these responses are linked. Conceptually, this hypothesis aligns with an evolving shift in thinking away from the starkly reductionist "piece by piece" biology of the past and toward the deeply aggregated "everything is connected" way of looking at physiology, anatomy, and behavior. A shift in electrical activity in one region would inescapably impact the presence of inflammation in another, which in turn would have some level of impact on oxygenation, which in turn has an effect on the neuronic activity that impacts mental health, and so on, with endless permutations across the "system of systems" that is the human body. This might help explain why cryotherapy seems to have a logarithmic effect on spastic disorders and mental health, in which improvements in one area are functionally associated with improvements in another—and it aligns well with our hypothesis that right-away improvements in one area of wellness beget improvements in others.

Recently, a complementary view has emerged to the "system of systems" understanding of cryotherapy effects—one that suggests not only that any single impact is likely to give rise to another but also that there may be an upstream cause for many of the observed improvements, and especially those that accumulate over a lifetime. In this hypothesis, the process of aging itself can be impacted by cryotherapy.

The genesis of this idea is a simple observation: For decades it has been known that animals that live in colder environments tend to live a bit longer than those of the same species in warmer environments,[30] and this rule appears to apply equally to endothermic animals, like mammals, and ectotherms, like reptiles.[31]

For a long time, this was more of a "gee whiz" observation than guidance for a healthy life. That began to change in the late 2010s, as researchers began to focus on the ways in which brown adipose tissue gradually disappears as we age. Humans have two main types of fat, brown and white; brown fat carries more mitochondria and burns more energy than white fat. Babies are born with lots of brown fat, and it used to be thought that it pretty much all went away as we aged. When that happens, we lose a rich source of the cellular organelles that are responsible for the lion's share of energy production in our bodies. But recent research has shown that cold exposure activates mitochondrial action in these forms of fat, essentially making it act more youthful and giving us the ability to produce and sustain more of it.[32]

An important clue as to why that happens came in 2021, when a team led by Polish biologist Magdalena Więcek discovered that the levels of two types of signaling proteins known as sirtuins, which are involved in human metabolic regulation, were increased in the bloodstreams of both athletically active and non-athletic but otherwise healthy men. That finding has ignited a flurry of other, ongoing research, because many scientists suspect sirtuins play a role in regulating the aging process, especially when exposed to a variety of stresses, in response to which they signal cells to slow reproduction and instead focus on maintenance and repair—a process that assures longer-term survival of those cells and the organisms they comprise.[33]

A lot of work would need to be done before anyone could say with any degree of scientific certainty that cryotherapy slows aging, but the holistic nature of its effects—coupled with early research into the molecular mechanisms that might impact upstream aging—make this a promising avenue for exploration.

In the meantime, a lot of clients have told us that the desire to limit biological aging is one of the key drivers of their decision to engage in regular cryotherapy.

"I'd say that aging is my key focus, and I do a lot to fight against it," Lanna, a professional musician in Venice Beach, California, told us. "One of the things that I've had to accept with this is that because aging is such a slow process and everyone goes through it differently, it's hard to say with absolute confidence that, yes, this one thing or that one thing is slowing down my rate of aging."

But Lanna said the myriad immediate and sustained effects she has felt since starting a weekly cryotherapy regimen have compelled upon her a strong belief that she is growing more well across the board. "And that, to me, points to aging," she said.

We do recognize that's all far less exciting and a lot more complicated than saying that "cryo slows aging." And in the long run we might all look back and wonder why it was that we weren't willing to be more bullish about this putative association. The increasing availability and affordability of epigenetic assessments of aging in coming years may help bring this revelation about sooner. But the key to this period of transition—in which the assumptions we've long made about what human health is and what health care should be are quickly changing—is applying what we know in measured ways, balancing what we've learned with an appreciation for all the unknowns, and then making the best decisions we can. Especially as it pertains to cryotherapy, we can make those decisions knowing that even if we don't yet understand all the potential benefits, decades of research and millions of experiences have demonstrated that the risks are low and the right-away benefits are high.

Cold Therapy at Home

We are confident that cryotherapy will soon be among the most widely used health interventions in the world, and that we will reach that future not decades upon decades from now, but in just a matter of years. Indeed, we think that future is long overdue.

In the meantime, though, it's important to consider what people can do if they don't yet have access to a place like Restore, where they can find a well-designed whole-body cryo chamber. That may provide the best possible experience, but there are lots of other ways to introduce the power of cold therapy into your life even if you never come to know what negative 150 degrees feels like on your entire body, all at once.

Your shower is the best starting place for this exploration. For a lot of people, the biggest obstacle to a cold shower is the idea of stepping directly into a stream of icy water, but there's no reason why you shouldn't start with whatever temperature you're used to and "slow roll" your way to a colder finish. Eventually, aiming for a period of several minutes—similar to the timeframe most people spend in a cryo chamber—is a worthwhile goal, but if at first you can only abide a "hot completely off" shower for 15 seconds, then you should celebrate those 15 seconds!

You should also take stock of how your body and mind feel after that experience. Take note of the areas where you frequently experience aches and pains. Roll your shoulders, shake your hips, and curl and extend your arms and legs. Gaze at a piece of art or look in the mirror: Does your mind feel clearer? Assess your mood: How are you doing? If you're like most people, even a short cold shower will offer a burst of energy—capacity that you can leverage for another health-promoting activity.

Mitchell, for instance, always tries to take a few minutes to meditate after he steps out of a cold shower.

"I've always believed in and benefited from meditation, but in my mind it had always been a practice I associated with sleep, sort of like a quick nap, and my thoughts during this time felt foggy," he said. "I just figured that was what meditation was supposed to feel like. But when I started meditating right after a cold shower, it was a different experience. My mind feels light and my thoughts feel crisp. When I would do what I now call 'sleepy meditation,' my ideas would drift, which can be a lovely experience but it's not necessarily great if your goal is to experience mindfulness. When I meditate after a cold shower I can hold on to an idea, something very specific, for a very long time, and it doesn't float away. I can examine it and appreciate it. I never knew what people meant when they'd say 'be one' with something. But now I really think I do."

For Mitchell, a quick cold shower builds capacity for meditation, which in turn builds capacity for combatting a common struggle—getting out of bed bright and early in the morning. "I used to hit my snooze button several times every day," he said. "I'd heard that the sleep I was getting in those extra minutes wasn't actually helpful, but I couldn't help myself. But it was shortly after I began this little trick of meditation after a cold shower that I realized that I wasn't nearly so tempted to reset my alarm. I felt so much more rested."

In 2015, researchers in the Netherlands recruited more than 3,000 people between the ages of 18 and 65 who weren't already habitual cold shower-takers and assigned them to various groups that would either shower normally or begin their bathing routine with hot water and finish up with at least 30 seconds of cold water. The result? Those who finished up with a "cold snap" were far less likely to miss work due to sickness. They also reported a better quality of life, improved work productivity, and decreased anxiety.[34]

What's better than a shower? Perhaps a complete dip. While a full ice bath or specially designed plunge tub may be out of reach for most people, unwarmed water from a home tap generally hovers between 45 and 55 degrees Fahrenheit, and just a couple trays of ice cubes from your freezer can buy another 5 degrees toward a colder goal. Is colder better? Almost certainly—especially if you want this to be an in-and-out experience—but studies of people immersed in 57-degree water for an hour have shown decreases in body temperature, increases in heart rate, and a 350 percent boost in metabolic rate, among other effects, including reduced stress hormones levels.[35] It doesn't take almost-ice conditions to introduce a profound cold response.

Likewise, it doesn't take a large swing in ambient temperatures to introduce our bodies to the sorts of temporary stresses that appear to be at the heart of the health benefits of cryotherapy. As many American soldiers who have served in the often brutally hot environments of the Middle East can attest, a 10- or 15-degree drop in temperature from 110 to 95 when the sun sinks over the desert horizon can induce a surprising and bizarre sense of frigidness. That's because our bodies seek homeostasis in all sorts of conditions—and once we've grown used to something, a little change can feel dramatic.

It's for this reason that it's likely beneficial to step into a very cold room after being outside on a very hot day, and why it's likely good for us to leave the warm confines of our homes on a very cold day. And while hypothermia is obviously a step too far, an hour of exercise in near-freezing temperature can do wonders, especially by helping transform energy-storing white fat into calorie-burning darker fats.

The bottom line is that while decades of innovation have given us better and better ways to administer cold therapy—and well-designed whole-body cryo is an experience that we believe everyone should have access to—the right-away impact of this modality can literally be obtained *right away*. This is, after all, a therapy older than Hippocrates himself. Back then, of course, the coldest conceivable temperatures were winter weather extremes, and while the Grecian mountains get a good cover of snow, most of that country rarely dips below freezing, so Hippocrates utilized cold water baths, which he proposed as an essential part of bringing the human body back into balance in times of sickness or injury.

This is, after all, a therapy older than Hippocrates himself.

There's some sad irony in this history. The power of this right-away intervention has been known for millennia, and yet few people consider getting cold to be healthful—most of us avoid it at all costs.

But it's time to reclaim what we never should have lost. It's time to get shivering. Right away.

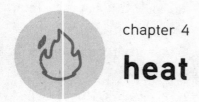

chapter 4

heat

A fter earning a bachelor's degree in Slavic languages and literature in the late 1990s, Jennifer Davis-Flynn knew where she wanted to be. The writer and amateur jazz vocalist packed up for Russia and spent the next eight years writing, singing, and making friends from all over the world in Saint Petersburg.

On Friday nights, Jennifer and her girlfriends would frequent a sauna in Liteyny Prospekt, a hip downtown thoroughfare where they'd share drinks and dish out the details of their lives.

"Saunas inspire naked truths," she would later write.[1]

But after returning to the United States, where saunas just aren't as *populyarnyy,* Jennifer fell out of the habit—until the early 2020s, when a local spa offered two months of unlimited infrared sauna visits for just under $200.

Up to six times a week, Jennifer would step into the sauna room, "turn on a podcast, and sink into the experience." After 30 days of this regular practice, her results were, well, *mixed.*

Some of the benefits she experienced were in line with the myriad claims that many sauna users espouse. "My skin looks better than it has in years," she noted, adding that she had also experienced "relief from chronic pain" and "a reduction in stress." She was disappointed, though, that all that constant sweating didn't result in any weight loss and didn't raise her heart rate any higher than about the level of a brisk walk.

The spa Jennifer went to had suggested that the experience would be life-changing. And against that standard, who could help but feel a little disappointed?

As you know, though, the virtuous cycle isn't about feeling better in *every way*. It's about feeling better *right away*. And that was Jennifer's experience. Her skin looked better. Her pain—from plantar fasciitis that had been bugging her for more than decade—had subsided. And she was feeling a lot less stressed. "I always leave feeling refreshed and inspired," she noted.

Expectations are important. When they're set too low, we're prone to indifference. When they're set too high, we're likely to experience disappointment. But in the exact same way that cold exposure can be beneficial to just about everyone in some way—and almost no one in the same way, let alone in every way—the benefits of heat-related therapies, which are backed by centuries of experience and many decades of solid, scientific research, hit everyone differently. So, this chapter is about helping you set your expectations just right when it comes to the spectrum of research-based benefits of heat-related treatments and therapies. Because while it's possible that this modality can indeed be life-changing all by itself, it's far more likely that it—like cryotherapy and the other steps we will introduce along the way—will represent a palpable, right-away step *toward* that goal.

It's also a step that many hundreds of millions of people have taken both as a cultural practice and with the explicit intention of seeking wellness.

We know some of the history of sauna from a comprehensive medical text written by the Roman encyclopedist Aulus Cornelius Celsus, who was plying his trade around the same time as Jesus of Nazareth was making his way around another part of the empire. In Celsus's medical guide, it was suggested that bodily swelling could be treated with heated sand or warm baths,[2] thus whole-body heat as a health-oriented therapy is at the very least about 2,000 years old.

In Finland, where sauna (pronounced in Finnish such that the first syllable rhymes with "cow") is such a ubiquitous cultural practice that there are more saunas than cars, the health benefits of this habit have been accepted as a matter of conventional wisdom for hundreds if not thousands of years. But in the past few decades, as sauna grew in popularity in other places in the world, the demand was also growing for actual medical evidence of the benefits most Finns took for granted.

Much of that evidence has indeed come from Finland, where surveys show that nearly everyone takes at least one sauna bath a week and many people sauna as often as every day. This has created a nearly ideal situation for studying the long-term impacts of sauna and the differing health effects that come from regularity of use. The one big challenge researchers have had to overcome is finding enough people who *don't* sauna to constitute a strong control group. Increasingly, though, this research is also being conducted in other parts of the world, and other cultural contexts, like Native American sweat lodges and Japanese onsen baths, offering more opportunities to see the benefits of heat exposure applied in different ways. And the good news is that there's nothing magical about one kind of heat therapy over another. Some are better in some ways, others are better in other ways, but nearly universally, these studies have demonstrated that heat can be an effective treatment for myriad conditions.

We are also starting to better understand why, and we'll take a deep dive into the answer to that question soon, but for the moment it suffices to say that as is the case in cryotherapy, heat exposure in safe conditions is a "good stress" that alters the expression of many genes in ways that are beneficial to our holistic health,[3] offering capacity we can reinvest into the virtuous cycle.

And that all starts with our hearts.

Warm-Hearted

The Kuopio Ischaemic Heart Disease Risk Factor Study wasn't intended to identify the benefits of sauna on health—no more so than the study was intended to help us better understand the consequences of drinking fermented milk, eating smoked salmon for breakfast, working odd hours, or feeling hopeless. But those are just some of the things we better understand today thanks to this longitudinal study, which was launched in the mid-1980s in the city of Kuopio in Eastern Finland, in which thousands of middle-aged men were asked hundreds of questions about their lives and lifestyles. And since a few of those questions were about sauna bathing—and the men have been checked in on at various times over the intervening decades—researchers have been able to identify many ways in which heat exposure impacts long-term health, and especially cardiovascular health.

Among the researchers who have been central to these discoveries is Jari Laukkanen, a jovial cardiologist who strives to make sure his work isn't just academic but actually applicable to people's lives. Laukkanen has authored or co-authored more than 400 studies on human health and, since the mid-2010s, much of that research has emerged from the data gathered in the Kuopio study and additional examinations of hospitalization and death records in Eastern Finland.

The first paper that Laukkanen and his colleagues published on this topic, in 2015, shocked many people—and even surprised many people in Finland who, as we've noted, had long assumed that sauna was good for their health but were taken aback by data that demonstrated a profound dose-response benefit. That analysis showed that in the first 20 years of the Kuopio study, the men who used a sauna with the greatest frequency were far less likely to suffer from sudden cardiac death, fatal coronary heart disease, and fatal cardiovascular disease. The amount of time the men spent in a sauna during each session mattered, too—the more, the better.[4]

There are, of course, plenty of factors that could be at play in this association. Even in Finland, where saunas abound, people with greater income have greater access to this part of cultural life, and people with more leisure time can enjoy it more than people who do not—and both money and leisure are monumental factors in health. But the analyses considered all that and more! The researchers adjusted for socioeconomic status as well as age, body mass index, blood pressure, cholesterol, smoking habits, alcohol consumption, previously diagnosed diseases, and physical activity. Among every subgroup, the benefits on heart health were affirmed, and follow-up studies have reaffirmed those benefits again and again.

Because the initial Kuopio subjects were all men, Laukkanen's team next focused on women. Using decades of surveys and records from 850 women from Kuopio and some of its nearby rural communities, the researchers repeated the steps they'd taken with the earlier cohort. The women's results didn't just mirror what had been seen in the men—they improved on them. More regular sauna use was associated with even fewer cardiovascular disease outcomes in women than in men who were assessed during the same years.[5]

In 2018, Laukkanen's group took another step toward explaining the profound cardiovascular benefits they were seeing in sauna users when they had 100 test subjects—about half men and half women—take a sauna in specific, controlled conditions: 163 degrees Fahrenheit at 10 to 20 percent humidity for 30 minutes. As the study participants stepped out of the sauna, they were subjected to tests for heart rate, arterial stiffness, and blood pressure, and their blood was drawn for further analysis. The result showed that on average, the half-hour sauna had raised people's heart rates similar to what they would have experienced at the end of a session of medium-intensity exercise, and that their blood pressure had been reduced. The most interesting change to the researchers, though, was that the subjects showed significant improvements in vascular compliance, the measurement of a blood vessel's ability to accommodate increased blood flow, a good indicator of heart health, since reduced compliance has been associated with heart failure.[6]

Of course, no one is going to notice improved heart health as an immediately perceptible benefit of a sauna visit. So while this is all good news, it's not a palpable step on the feel-better-do-more cycle. But that's OK, because there are plenty of other ways in which heat exposure may help you feel better right away.

Mental and Cognitive Health

One of the reasons why few people in Finland had even felt the need for proof of quantifiable health benefits of sauna is because they knew very well, from personal experience, that heat exposure left them feeling relaxed, refreshed, alert, and overall more healthy.

"Maybe you couldn't put your finger exactly on what it was that felt so good about sauna," said Torben, who grew up in Helsinki and moved to Austin to attend graduate school in his mid-20s, "but to me, it was like good sleep. If I didn't have an opportunity for sauna for many days in a row, I felt much worse, and I knew this was unhealthy. When I did maintain my regular pattern, I felt much better."

These days, however, it's not just vague feelings that attest to the right-away power of sauna. Researchers have found that the feelings of relaxation associated with sauna are also linked to a nearly immediate increase in the production of circulating endorphins, the natural chemical signalers that block the perception of pain and increase the sensation of well-being.[7] These hormone responses don't last long—they return to normal levels not long after the experience is over—but that short period of mitigated pain and accentuated well-being can be reinvested into other actions to amplify the psychological gains.[8]

Torben, for instance, is among a growing number of people who have taken to using a sauna before they exercise—not after, as many people do, as a reward for a good workout. "There are probably benefits both ways," he said. "But I have found that the good feelings I get from sauna are a big help for me, since I honestly am not the biggest fan of exercise to begin with. It sort of helps get me going."

And after that, he said, the exercise endorphins kick in. "And the cool thing that happens at that point is that I feel this rush of happiness and satisfaction, and it's even jacked up by the fact that I know what happens when I exercise," he said. "It means I'm going to sleep well, and I know that's going to make me feel better, too, so it's really a lovely sort of chain reaction."

In the longer term, what Torben calls a "chain reaction," and what we see as part of the virtuous cycle, is fantastic for our brains. Using the Kuopio population study group, Laukkanen and his team identified hundreds of people who over the course of many decades suffered from various sorts of mental health disorders. Compared to those who used a sauna at least four times per week, those who only had one session per week were four times more likely to have been diagnosed with one of these conditions.[9]

"It's really a lovely sort of chain reaction."

Emerging evidence suggests mental health disorders experienced earlier in life increase the risk for dementia later on.[10] As such, it might not be surprising that among the Kuopio cohort, those who used sauna more often throughout their lives were far less likely to develop Alzheimer's and other dementias.[11]

There is still a lot of work that needs to be done to understand these associations, including the mechanistic reasons why sauna appears to have such profound benefits for mental health and long-term brain health. There are also plenty of questions left to be resolved as to whether these associations will hold up in longitudinal studies of people outside of Finland. And while there is plenty of reason to believe that they will, much of that evidence is unlikely to materialize in the near future. After all, the Finns began their efforts to study the residents of Kuopio many decades ago; similar data collection efforts are only now beginning in many places in the world, or haven't even gotten started.

It's going to be important for researchers to evaluate the ways in which the most common Finnish ways of using sauna—hot, dry, and often—produce results that are similar and different to heat therapies in other contexts, like wet saunas, lower-temperature saunas, home baths, and communal hot baths.

Laukkanen thinks it's likely. "We have not compared different types of saunas and their health effects. Our studies are based on hot and dry saunas," he told us. But, he said, those other forms of heat therapy "may offer similar effects to a typical Finnish sauna."

The effort to know for sure feels especially important to us for several reasons.

First, while the saunas we've made available to our communities at Restore centers across North America are similar in many ways to the saunas commonly found in Finland, they are also different in some ways, chiefly that the saunas you find in Finland are most often heated with wood-fired stoves or electric heaters, which heat the air inside the space, whereas we've chosen to provide our clients with an infrared sauna experience, the latter of which heats the body more directly, and potentially more penetratingly, even though it doesn't warm up the surrounding air as much. This is more energy efficient and is less of a potential fire hazard, but there are plenty of advocates of the "tried and true" Finnish methods, and we respect that.

Second, even if our loftiest ambitions are realized in the near future and many others follow along in providing accessible and affordable sauna experiences within a short distance of every home, everywhere, we would still exist in a world that's a far cry away from the ubiquity of sauna availability in Finland, so knowing which alternative experiences work, as well, will help ensure that more people can benefit.

Finally, and put simply, we cannot imagine anything more important than psychological and cognitive health, without which there is no point in any other types of health. Thus, the faster we can arrive in a world in which the weight of scientific evidence establishes that other forms of heat therapy can have similar effects to those that have been observed in Finland, the better.

That work is underway. In the meantime, however, we should not stop at the benefits to cardiovascular and cognitive health. There's so much more.

Heat and Pain

Although it was cryotherapy that drew us into the world of wellness, it took no time at all for us to recognize that the principle of right-away wellness that we saw as such a game-changing aspect of cryo also existed in other therapies—interventions that, for whatever reason, have not been adopted more widely in mainstream health care settings. And since cold drew us into this world, we suppose it makes sense that heat would be the next logical thing to look at, particularly given the long history of success and research related to sauna.

But while the longitudinal data was interesting and exciting to us, what was most pertinent to our decision on whether to offer sauna as another wellness modality in our centers was whether we could establish that the infrared saunas that appear to be the best fit for those centers could indeed offer a meaningful right-away benefit to our customers. And that's why we zeroed in on pain. After all, it can take a long time—decades of longitudinal research—to know whether an intervention is having an impact on long-term states of physical and mental wellness and disease. But pain is different; we can know whether an intervention like infrared heat therapy can influence acute pain in literal minutes.

One of the first well-controlled studies to offer some potential answers to this question came from a team of researchers in Japan who were studying a form of treatment called waon, or "soothing warmth" therapy, which had been developed by a cardiologist named Chuwa Tei. Tei's unconventional method of treating patients with various heart conditions included time in an infrared sauna, which he chose based on the notion that the radiant energy created by infrared heating devices would be more penetrating than a traditional sauna. What is interesting about the waon study is that the research team wasn't initially interested in whether this experimental therapy was useful for mitigating pain. What they wanted to know was whether the therapy was having an impact on various forms of heart disease. But in a study of mice they became aware that infrared exposure appeared to be alleviating pain in animals with heart conditions that were causing an inadequate blood supply to their legs, and having seen this in mice, they decided that they needed to investigate it in people, too. When they did, in a group of 21 people who were treated for six weeks with infrared sauna treatments, they noted a significant decrease in reports of leg pain.[12]

At about the same time, thousands of miles away in the Netherlands, a team of researchers specializing in rheumatoid arthritis and ankylosing spondylitis were investigating the effects of twice-a-week infrared sauna treatments over the course of a month. After each therapy session, the researchers noted, the test subjects reported less pain and stiffness, and over the course of the study they noted a trend toward accumulating beneficial effects.[13]

These studies are both good news because the results are similar to those that have been observed in traditional Finnish saunas[14]—and, importantly, in some different cultural settings.

It would be fair to ask whether we're cherry-picking the data here.

After all, we've invested in infrared saunas. So, we'd like to make something clear: Saunas of any kind aren't likely the only way to achieve these results. If you have a bathtub and a good water heater, you can likely experience many of the benefits that are associated with sauna with a good, long, hot soak.

That was Kaylee's experience after she broke multiple bones in her leg in a ski accident a few years ago. As she began the long and painful process toward recovery, her physical therapist was adamant that she should precede her rehabilitative exercises by soaking her leg in a hot bath. "I'd sit there for 10 or 15 minutes," she told us, "and it definitely decreased my pain and helped me to relax. After that I could do about an hour of exercise."

"The difference is huge," she told us. "When I don't do it—if I forget or don't have time—I can't exercise as much. And when I do it, I feel much better for longer, and I get more exercise in."

More exercise meant faster improvements. For Kaylee, faster improvements meant walking, then running, and then eventually skiing again. These days, she's back on the slopes in the winter and, during the summers, she's running around the soccer field with the high school players she coaches. Her story isn't unusual. It's no secret among physical therapists that hot water immersion is a right-away intervention that builds capacity through pain relief. It likely has many other impacts as well on both mental and physical health, which is why we strongly believe that a good, long soak in a hot bath—110 degrees Fahrenheit or so, which is hot enough to prompt a physiological response but not generally hot enough to burn the skin—is a great way to access the power of this element of hyper wellness. And yet there just aren't a lot of studies on hot water immersion for physical therapy, let alone other health conditions, in no small part because funding such studies isn't easy. After all, there's nothing to sell on the other end—just a better life.

And likely a longer one, too.

A Heated Discussion on Aging

In the early 2010s, researchers from the Onsen Medical Science Research Center at Tokyo's Japan Health and Research Institute wanted to know whether hot spring baths might be a force multiplier for other healthy practices—and to begin their exploration of that question they centered on another common Japanese practice.

They knew that catechin—a compound known for its potent antioxidant properties—was one of the reasons that green tea appears to have such significant health benefits.[15] So, they set up an experiment in which some onsen users would drink tea before entering the hot spring and then have a small amount of blood drawn, while others drank tea but didn't take an onsen bath and simply waited for the same amount of time before having a sample taken. When they compared the samples, they found that plasma levels of catechin were higher in those who had followed up the tea with a plunge in a hot spring.[16]

What's causing this sort of reaction? That's hard to say—not because we don't know what changes in the body when our internal temperature rises as a result of temporary heat exposure, like that which happens in a sauna or hot bath, but because there are so many different things that happen all at once. This is called pleiotropy, a phenomenon that occurs when myriad and often unrelated systems are affected by a single stimulus. Researchers have not yet concluded what happens first, second, third, and so on. But when we expose ourselves to heat for relatively short durations (as little as a few minutes, and under an hour in almost all cases to avoid dehydration and other potential problems, although there are many factors at play, including how the heat is applied and how hot it is), here are just some of the things[17] we know are happening:

First, there are the processes and conditions that are reduced as a result of heat immersion. That includes low-density lipoprotein cholesterol, which is often called "bad" cholesterol, as well as triglycerides, a type of fat in our blood that the body uses for energy but that, at high levels, can cause heart attacks. Arterial stiffness is also reduced by heat exposure, as is intimal medial thickness, which is a measurement of the thickness of the inside lining of our arteries. Likely as a result of all this, blood pressure tends to fall. Inflammation also tends to decrease as a result of heat exposure, as do levels of reactive oxygen species, a type of molecule that can damage DNA.

And then there are the processes that are increased as a result of heat immersion. High-density lipoprotein—the "good" blood particles that absorb cholesterol and carry it back to the liver—gets a boost. So does arterial compliance, the measurement of an artery's ability to accommodate increased blood flow. The function of endothelial cells, which govern the opening and closing of arteries and control levels of fluids and electrolytes in our blood, is also improved during heat exposure. Endothelial cells also produce nitric oxide, a naturally occurring gas that relaxes blood vessels and increases blood flow when our body temperatures rise. Owing to all this, overall cardiorespiratory fitness, which is the capacity of the circulatory and respiratory systems to supply oxygen to our energy-producing mitochondria, is increased. And likely related, although in a chicken-and-egg mystery that no one has solved just yet, is an increase in the function of the immune system.

There's more. But you undoubtedly have gotten the gist of what's happening. Some studies show more profound effects. Others show more tempered reactions. But there doesn't seem to be any research that indicates any process that doesn't fit the pattern of "bad stuff" getting muted and "good stuff" getting accentuated.

Whenever we see these sorts of broad, pleiotropically beneficial patterns, it's a good indication that whatever stimulus is at play isn't acting individually on each disparate biological system, but may in fact be putting pressure on the "master switch" of wellness: aging.

That's what Rhonda Patrick appears to suspect is happening. While many people know her as the host of a popular health podcast, Patrick got her start as a cell biologist—and she still publishes in peer-reviewed journals, including a 2021 paper on the health impacts of sauna. In that report, Patrick ticked off a list of beneficial short- and long-term physiological responses to heat stress, and in nearly every one, she made note of the connection to biological aging. "Sauna bathing," she wrote, "may offer a means to forestall the effects of aging and extend healthspan."[18]

Stacking the Contrasts

To Patrick, the beneficial impacts of sauna are all about hormesis, the body's all-hands-on-deck response to a mild stressor, which which sets off a protective response within our cells to repair damage and provide protection from future threats, whether real or perceived, that may be even stronger.

Exercise is a hormetic stressor. Cold is, too. And we can add heat to that list as well. Patrick has spoken extensively about the benefits of all these stressors—and of using them in conjunction with one another, a practice that many people call "stacking," which we've come to see as a turbocharger of the virtuous cycle.

Indeed, many of our clients have integrated contrast therapy—heat and cold in close succession—into their personal wellness regimen. Contrast therapy has been demonstrated to increase blood flow and oxygenation of muscle tissue,[19] as well as lessen muscle soreness and improve muscle strength recovery after exercise.[20]

"I feel like it's the secret sauce of what I've been doing here," Jonah, a client from San Diego told us after a session that began with cryotherapy and ended with a sauna bath. "I get different things from both these therapies. Cryo has been a big help with my psoriasis, and sauna definitely helps me with sleep restlessness. But when it comes to my mental state—like being clear and focused and also feeling happy—whenever I do contrast it's like being on a different level."

"I feel like it's the secret sauce of what I've been doing here."

Harvard geneticist David Sinclair is another advocate of contrast therapy—a practice that he has integrated into workouts with his teenaged son. Sinclair has proposed that stacking these elements helps trigger the ancient and well-conserved genes that control aging in nearly every life form. "Hormesis is generally good for organisms, especially when it can be induced without causing any lasting damage," he wrote in 2019. "When hormesis happens, all is well. And, in fact, all is better than well, because the little bit of stress that occurs when the genes are activated prompts the rest of the system to hunker down, to conserve, to survive a little longer. That's the start of longevity."[21]

Great Expectations

In Sinclair's view, if a hormetic stress is having an effect on aging—the upstream driver of nearly every disease—then it should be observable across nearly all areas of health.

Indeed, researchers have found that heat therapy is associated with a lower risk of dementia and Alzheimer's.[22] It also appears to reduce the risk of infectious diseases,[23] respiratory diseases,[24] and stroke.[25] And it has been associated with significant reductions in inflammation and oxidative stress across a person's lifetime.[26]

So, when we learned of a study in which the impacts of heat therapy—specifically the Finnish style of sauna bathing—were investigated in relation to the risk of cancer, we expected it would demonstrate a similarly beneficial impact. That's what the authors, who were working with the longitudinal health data from Kuopio, seem to have expected to see as well. They didn't. There was in fact no difference at all in the cancer rates of people who used sauna often and those who used it infrequently.[27]

We think this finding is important for several reasons. First, it came from the same group of Finnish researchers, led by cardiologist Laukkanen, who have been responsible for so many other findings of the health benefits of sauna. Over decades of building businesses, we've learned that if someone is only ever telling you what you expect to hear—and, even more, what you want to hear—you're probably not getting the full story. So, while Laukkanen's cancer study didn't reveal an expected result, let alone a positive result, the result for us was increased confidence in his team's research in general. Second, it's a reminder that while the hormetic stress hypothesis about holistic aging is compelling, it's still a hypothesis that will need many more years of further exploration, in many more settings. We're bullish about this hypothesis, but excitement isn't a substitute for good, sound science—and science takes time. Third, it's a reflection of the fact that the human body is a complicated "system of systems," and when dealing with such complexity, we shouldn't expect magic-bullet solutions to all problems.

What, then, can we say with a tremendous amount of certainty right now? Well, when it comes to heat exposure, we can say a lot. We know, for instance, that it offers quick and palpable benefits for pain and mobility, and that many people feel it has an immediate and profound impact on their mental health. That's the start of capacity—the central currency of the feel-better-do-more cycle. That alone might explain the long-term health benefits associated with the hot and dry model of Finnish sauna specifically and heat immersion more generally, but there is also reason to suspect that the hormetic stress that comes with exposing our bodies to such conditions is acting on upstream drivers of many different diseases, and perhaps aging itself.

In the end, though, what matters most is your experience. Does heat immersion—however derived—give you an immediately palpable sense of improved well-being? Are you able to reinvest that right-away benefit into the virtuous cycle? If so, heat exposure should be a regular part of the habits you maintain as you work toward hyper wellness.

But everybody is different. And that is the central reality that has driven our decision to build studios that offer people the opportunity to stack multiple therapies that work across the nine elements. Because if the holistic effect of two or more therapies is greater than the sum of the parts—and we've seen compelling evidence that this has been the case for many people—then giving our clients the ability to stack these interventions in a way that makes sense to them offers them the ability to feel *even* better, do *even* more, and thereby amplify the tailwinds that will help push them toward their hyper wellness goals.

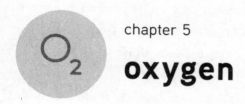

chapter 5

oxygen

At 7,700 feet above sea level, Addis Ababa is already one of the highest major cities in the world. But when you head north from the Ethiopian capital on Highway A3, through the serene and deeply green Entoto Natural Park, zigzagging across the invisible border that separates the city from the northern Oromia countryside, the road just keeps on going higher.

A few miles into that journey, there is an eastern bend in the highway, where you will find the Yaya Africa Athletics Village, a high-altitude training center cofounded by two-time Olympic gold medal distance runner Haile Gebrselassie. Since 2010, athletes from around the world have been coming to train at Yaya—some staying for weeks or months before dropping to lower elevations for high-impact training and races.

Jamal, who made his first visit to Yaya in 2017, was a long-time triathlete who had, in his mid-30s, begun to notice that he simply wasn't able to keep on improving on his tri performances the way he had for more than a decade. "I was never a top finisher or anything close," he said. "I always just ran against myself, always trying to better my own times, and for a long time I kept getting faster and stronger. Then I hit 35, and something just changed. And even though I knew that I would slow down eventually—because that's just how life goes—I wasn't ready for it to happen just yet."

Jamal had also been a long-time fan of British distance runner Mo

Farah, one of the most successful endurance athletes of all time. And after reading that Farah had trained at Yaya, Jamal asked his boss for permission to work abroad for a month and booked a trip to Ethiopia—the first he'd ever taken to the country his maternal grandfather had emigrated from in the 1950s. There, he met a lot of other athletes from around the world, from Olympic hopefuls to amateurs like himself—all hoping to take the next step in performance.

"At first, it was hard to run at that altitude," he said. "It took my body about a week to get used to it, and even then there was just no way I could go as fast and as far as I was used to."

But after growing accustomed to training at an altitude in which oxygen saturation was about 15 percent, returning to run at sea level—where oxygen saturation is nearly 21 percent—was a dream. "It was like having a superpower," Jamal said. "It's incredible how easy things feel when your body is getting more oxygen."

Sure enough, in the races that he completed in the wake of his stay in the Ethiopian mountains, Jamal charted his best performance in years. "Going to Africa to train was sort of a once-in-a-lifetime thing," he said. "But I fell in love with how my body felt when I would get a huge boost in the oxygen levels I'd grown accustomed to, so I found places closer to home where I could live at elevation for a while, and then I'd run at sea level and it made me feel so fantastic."

"It's incredible how easy things feel when your body is getting more oxygen."

Few of us spend as much time thinking about oxygen the way that Jamal does these days. But even (and perhaps especially) if we are not endurance athletes, we would all do well to spend more time considering what happens as oxygen passes from our alveoli to our capillaries, and from there into our red blood cells for transport into our hearts and distribution to the rest of the body, where it's taken in by all our other cells, which use it to produce energy.

Over time, our bodies are adept at getting the oxygen we need out of the atmosphere in which we live, which is why Jamal was able to get used to training at altitude during his month in Yaya and the other high-elevation cities where he now vacations. But increases in available oxygen, which lead to increased blood oxygen levels, can provide a boost of energy, clarity of thought, immunity, and recovery from exercise or injury, which is likely why Jamal initially feels superhuman whenever he returns to training and racing at sea level.

While some athletes have made "live high/run low" a key element of their lives—and studies have shown this practice can enhance exercise economy, blood flow, and performance[1]—it's not a practical way to achieve these sorts of benefits. And even if you already happen to live at elevation, have an easy route to much lower altitudes, and have all the time in the world to make the trek back and forth to take advantage of the difference in air pressure and oxygen saturation (and, by the way, we know nobody like this), the difference in O_2 is fractional.

But a fast-emerging and compelling body of research is demonstrating that the administration of hyperbaric oxygen—breathing pure oxygen in a pressurized environment—may mimic and even improve upon this tactic. And when we began searching for interventions that, like cryotherapy and sauna, could offer a right-away boost in wellness, we began to suspect that we, too, should start thinking more about the role and power of oxygen in our lives.

A Hyperbaric History Lesson

The fact that we breathe air, and cannot live without it, is self-evident. But it wasn't until the late 1700s that we had much of a clue as to the substances that make up that air. That discovery came thanks to Joseph Priestley, a British antimonarchist who happened to be a close friend of Benjamin Franklin, whose insatiable curiosity was fueled by a belief that scientific discovery would lead to the overthrow of the idea of divine authority and the royals who perpetuated it to maintain power.[2]

Of course, it was tea, taxation, and the alluring notion of liberty that ultimately led to the slow dismantling of the British empire, starting with the loss of the American colonies in 1783, but Priestley's isolation of oxygen, a substance he at first called "dephlogisticated air," would be every bit as world-changing, albeit in different ways, for it set into motion a complete transformation of the way we understood the sustenance of life. Oxygen, we would later come to learn, makes up about 21 percent of the atmosphere and is an essential element of the energy-producing chemistry that drives metabolism in most living things and, of course, in every human being. It might seem to stand to reason, then, that air that is more pressurized or more saturated in oxygen, or both, might be beneficial to our wellness, but it took centuries before we would understand how to safely and effectively bring that basic principle into our lives.

The idea that pressurized air could be beneficial to health is older than the discovery of oxygen itself—it can be traced back to another British polymath, a 17th-century physician named Nathaniel Henshaw, whose theories on such matters appear to have been rooted in intuition more than any actual science. But in the early part of the 20th century, as the biochemical function of oxygen became clear following Priestley's discoveries, the reasons that hyperbaric pressure might indeed be beneficial began to take shape, and pneumatic chambers were built by scientists, engineers, and physicians across Europe and North America for the treatment of conditions ranging from tuberculosis to whooping cough and from cholera to conjunctivitis, using fabricated metal chambers that could create pressures as great as four atmospheres—that's 400 percent of the average air pressure at sea level.

If that sounds dangerous to you, you're not wrong. These early chambers often malfunctioned and sometimes claimed the lives of the patients inside, or left them ill or injured in ways they hadn't been when they consented to this novel treatment in the first place. It didn't help matters that some hyperbaric experimenters and advocates, like the eccentric American physician Orval Cunningham, were guarded about sharing their methods and results. Cunningham declined to allow the Bureau of Investigation of the American Medical Association to investigate his work, leading to accusations of quackery and damaging the progress of hyperbaric medicine for generations to come.[3]

Progress on using hyperbaric pressure to treat various diseases never stalled out entirely, but until the mid-20th century, these chambers were designed for the treatment of decompression sickness, which is caused when gases inside the body form bubbles during a rapid shift from a state of compression, especially during underwater diving. Some decades before, a German mechanic named Heinrich Dräger had begun experimenting with compression in the building of a beer-tap system that used compressed carbon dioxide, and later developed a coffin-sized "recompression chamber" in an effort to help divers afflicted by "the bends." Building from this initial work, a series of innovators added steps, processes, and safety mechanisms such that, by the outbreak of World War II, hyperbaric oxygen was the go-to treatment for military and construction divers suffering from decompression. With hyperbaric chambers spread out in just about every coastal city in the world in the decades following that war, it was not unusual for researchers to begin wondering about what other medical applications hyperbaric oxygen might be used for, and a second wave of scientific interest began to emerge.

In the 1960s, researchers showed pressurized oxygen could be used to help treat infections like tetanus and gangrene,[4] was effective in treating carbon monoxide poisoning,[5] appeared to help reduce skeletal inflammation,[6] and was effective in helping victims of stroke.[7] In the 1970s, studies showed potential applications for hyperbaric oxygen in heart attacks[8] and brain injuries.[9] In the 1980s, scientists demonstrated that people treated with radiation therapy to the head and neck were less likely to suffer from osteoradionecrosis, a form of bone death, if they were quickly treated with hyperbaric oxygen.[10] Year by year, the evidence of the effectiveness of this form of treatment has continued to mount.

If you're beginning to wonder why there isn't a hyperbaric chamber in every doctor's office in your community, you're not alone. That's what we began to wonder as well, as we explored the history and current trajectory of hyperbaric oxygen treatment, which is often known by its acronym, HbOT.

If you're beginning to wonder why there isn't a hyperbaric chamber in every doctor's office in your community, you're not alone.

The obvious (albeit perhaps a bit conspiratorially minded) answer is that just like cryotherapy chambers and saunas, hyperbaric chambers can be sold once and stay in service for many decades with proper maintenance—there is little profit motive in interventions like this. A perhaps more generous assessment, however, would suggest that the first wave of hyperbaric exploration, and the therapy's loss of favor in the wake of Cunningham's rejection of the American Medical Association's investigations, coincided with an explosion in the development of effective pharmaceuticals, and that is simply the treatment option that gained the most steam during the last century.[11] Ultimately, both of these factors likely played a role.

But the reasons that so many people don't have access to HbOT matter less than what can be done about it today. And that's why we've worked hard to make hyperbaric treatment accessible across the nation.

The Softer Side of Hyperbaric Treatment

At the time we were exploring the possibility of providing access to hyperbaric oxygen therapy in our centers, the US Food and Drug Administration, which oversees the approval of medical treatments, had green-lighted hyperbaric oxygen for fourteen conditions: decompression sickness, carbon monoxide poisoning, wound healing, diabetic wounds, radiation injuries, burns, skin infections, skin grafts, bone infections, sudden hearing loss, air embolism, crush injuries, anemia, and vision loss.

But Scott Sherr, a California physician who specializes in hyperbaric therapy, explained to us that in other countries, hyperbaric oxygen is used for more than 70 additional conditions. This also echoed what we'd discovered about cold- and heat-immersion therapies, which had been successfully used to help people live better lives in other nations for decades but—for whatever reason—hadn't gained momentum in our home country. Sherr also told us that even people who were suffering from the FDA-listed conditions often could not access HbOT because of insurance barriers, a lack of chambers in their community, or a lack of knowledge about its benefits by their doctors.

At first, it seemed like the solution was simple and straightforward. But there were several obstacles in our way. Foremost was that there are a lot of regulations surrounding the building, sale, and commercial use of "hard" hyperbaric chambers. Those are the rigid, heavily reinforced chambers that can be brought up to pressures as high as six atmospheres, although 1.5 to 2.5 atmospheres are far more common levels for most treatments.

We're not fans of overregulation, but some of these rules do make sense. Oxygen is essential for fire, after all. This was the very quality that led Joseph Priestley to identify it as something different from the other "airs" he identified in the late 1700s. As such, pressurized, enriched oxygen environments are a mere spark away from disaster. In 1997, hyperbaric medicine pioneer Paul Sheffield estimated that at least 77 people had died in 35 hyperbaric chamber fires in the previous 75 years.[12] Today, such tragedies are rare, in no small part because most nations have indeed regulated the design and use of hyperbaric chambers. But we could see that the sheer cost and regulatory hurdles that surround HbOT were going to be hard to surmount and scale for use in our centers.

There was another option—so-called "soft" chambers that were designed to be portable and that had been approved by the FDA for altitude sickness. These devices are limited to about 1.5 atmospheres, with elevated but not total oxygen saturation, and are thus tremendously less prone to causing pressure damage or creating a risk of fire. They also didn't have more than a century of use and research behind them, though, and it wasn't at first clear that there were actual wellness benefits to be derived at the levels that soft chambers could achieve.

More research is still needed. But just as the eccentricities of inventors like Orval Cunningham seem to have adversely impacted the progress of hard-chamber science in the early 20th century, some of the pioneers of soft-chamber hyperbaric systems had opinions that were critical and even hostile to mainstream science. Their ideas about health and wellness were sometimes conceived in ways that were different from how most physicians and scientific researchers look at the world. For instance, Bruce and Judy McKeeman, who submitted an application to the FDA in 2007 to market a "portable mild hyperbaric chamber" for the purpose of treating altitude sickness, have explained that they conceived of the idea of a less expensive alternative to hard hyperbaric chambers when they learned that the oxygen content of Earth before the massive flood described early in the Hebrew scriptures was twice what it is today.[13] In fact, scientists have estimated that there was a period of time in which the planet's atmospheric oxygen content reached about 35 percent, although that occurred about 300 million years ago versus the flood said to have occurred in the time of Noah, which biblical accounts suggest happened about 4,300 years ago, when oxygen levels were little different than what they are today.[14] While scriptural and scientific history can coexist in many situations, such views nonetheless put people like the McKeemans out of step with mainstream doctors and researchers. So even as soft-chamber hyperbaric systems gained approval for altitude sickness, many scientists and physicians were reluctant to be associated with these systems, and the research progress and doctor-supervised use of soft chamber hyperbaric therapy may have been slowed as a result.

But while the FDA regulates the health claims that can be made by device manufacturers and marketers, it cannot stop average, ordinary people from sharing their own experiences with such devices. And that's what began happening in the 2010s when soft chambers manufactured by the McKeemans and others began making their way into the world. Most interesting to us were the endless reports of right-away impacts—from athletic recovery to reduced headaches to mitigation of pain—which we saw as an indication that soft-chamber hyperbaric therapies might play an important role in the virtuous cycle that leads us toward hyper wellness. As that anecdotal evidence mounted, some researchers have overcome their initial reluctance to investigate the impacts of what is now generally called "mild hyperbaric oxygen therapy," or mHbOT. It was on the strength of this collective evidence that we committed to extending hyperbaric oxygen to Restore users across the nation.

Since that time, in our centers, we've seen substantial evidence that mHbOT has many of the same impacts as decades of research have indicated can be derived from traditional forms of hyperbaric therapy. It's nonetheless of the utmost importance that we differentiate between these two modalities. In this chapter, when a study or experience is related to HbOT, we will say so. And when the research or anecdote is centered on mHbOT, we'll make note of that as well. We will trust you to decide for yourself what benefits you might derive from one, the other, or both of these approaches.

Here for the Long Haul

Tim thought he was over COVID. He had tested positive in December 2020 and, like most people, fought through a few days of misery before making what he thought was a full recovery. As a previously healthy and active person, he figured that was that.

But two months later, he was once again feeling awful.

"I got hit by some symptoms that were dizziness, fatigue, and really just unable to function for about three weeks. That's when I ran to the doctors and said, 'Hey, something's wrong with me. Can you help me?'"

The US Centers for Disease Control has estimated that about 1 in 5 adults who have had COVID wind up as "long haulers," meaning their symptoms perpetuate for months and even years after the virus is no longer detectable in their body. Researchers have identified four major subtypes of this condition, each of which is defined by different clusters of symptoms. Individuals in the group known as Subphenotype 2, for instance, often suffer from breathing difficulties.[15]

That was what Tim was experiencing. The lack of oxygen was causing headaches, dizziness, fatigue, and brain fog. "I'd be doing the dishes and forget where they go. We're driving down the road and I'd forget where I'm going with my kids in the car."

Tests showed that Tim was getting only about 50 percent of the oxygen he needed. But the drugs he was prescribed seemed to make things worse—taking away his ability to sleep and speak.

At that point, Tim couldn't even walk the length of his home without gasping for breath. Fearing he would die if he couldn't find a treatment that would work to restore the oxygen in his body, Tim found his way to a Restore center in Chesterfield, Missouri, about 30 minutes from his home, where he had his first experience with mHbOT. After just one session in the soft chamber, Tim perceived a noticeable difference in his ability to breathe and speak.

The impact lasted just two hours. But after four months of suffering, those two hours felt like a miracle. So Tim returned, again and again, and with each session his ability to breathe improved. "By the seventh session, I could go a whole day and just feel great," he said.

And this part is important: Tim didn't just revel in his newfound ability to breathe again. He reinvested that tailwind into building even more capacity—walking, then riding a bike, then jogging, then running. And a month after his first hyperbaric session, he participated in a 5K.

"I ended up taking third," he said. "I couldn't walk 100 feet a month prior."

Around the same time Tim was being treated with mHbOT in Missouri, a team of scientists and physicians from University Hospital Coventry and Warwickshire in the United Kingdom gathered 10 long-haul COVID sufferers and treated them with 10 HbOT sessions over 12 days. In a peer-reviewed article in *Clinical Medicine*, a journal published by the Royal College of Physicians, the researchers reported "large" improvements in cognition, executive function, and verbal function, and "very large" improvements in attention, information processing, and the reduction of fatigue. "The mechanism of long COVID is still uncertain," the researchers wrote, noting that one common hypothesis is that many symptoms are the result of inadequate oxygen to maintain tissue function. "This is frequently the common denominator for many diseases that are responsive to HbOT." So while their study was small, with just 10 participants and no control group, the researchers wrote that pressurized oxygen supplementation was "a highly promising intervention."[16]

As further evidence that many physicians weren't waiting for larger studies to help their patients recover from COVID, a team of doctors from the Georgetown University School of Medicine wrote in 2021 that they were observing a huge influx of patients at hyperbaric centers that had been used for decades for wound care. The new admissions were so numerous that the wound-care doctors expressed concern that their patients might not be able to get the treatment they needed.[17] And this was in an environment in which hyperbaric therapy hadn't been approved by federal medical authorities for COVID treatment. The doctors were essentially prescribing this treatment "off label," in such numbers that it was threatening to overwhelm the existing system.

We also saw this wave of referrals at Restore centers across the nation, as long haulers who either couldn't access HbOT or whose insurance wouldn't pay for it came to our centers seeking mHbOT on the advice of their physicians. And again and again the staff members in our centers witnessed transformative changes like what Tim had experienced.

The doctors were essentially prescribing this treatment "off label," in such numbers that it was threatening to overwhelm the existing system.

Although the worst days of the pandemic are receding into the past, we still have many clients who are dealing with symptoms of long COVID. But word of the effectiveness of hyperbaric treatment on the symptoms of that disease also appears to be opening people's minds to other possibilities, in ways that are changing their lives for the better.

Mental Health

If you've ever filled your car's tires using a coin-operated air pump at a service station, you know that as long as the machine is operating properly and the hose is long enough, you can usually fill up all four tires in just a few minutes. And if you've ever tried to fill those same tires with a hand-operated bicycle pump, you also know that it takes a long time and a whole lot of effort. These two kinds of pumps don't differ much in terms of the pressure they create—100 pounds per square inch is fairly standard—but one creates constant air pressure while the other offers bursts of air pressure. And while it's a bit of a crude analogy, the pressure that exists outside our bodies works the same way to fill our lungs. The more pressure there is, and the more constant it is, the easier it is for us to breathe, not just because our lungs must do less work in creating the pressure differential to draw air in, but because the added pressure is essentially "smushing" the oxygen molecules into the openings of our alveoli, the microscopic air sacs in which oxygen is exchanged for carbon dioxide.

The air pressure at sea level is usually somewhere around 14.7 pounds per square inch. At that pressure, we must actively draw breath into our bodies by expanding our lungs, creating a vacuum that draws the air inward. Since we don't all live at sea level, though, on average the pressure is a little less. At 1,000 feet above sea level (such as Atlanta, Georgia), pressure hovers around 14.2 psi. At 2,000 feet (that's San Jose, California), it's 13.7 psi. At 3,000 feet (Tucson, Arizona), it's 13.2, and so on up to places like Breckenridge, Colorado, at 10,000 feet above sea level, where air pressure hovers around 10.1 pounds per square inch. As a result, many of us are working just a little bit harder than our friends in Miami, New York, San Diego, and other sea-level cities around the world, who are benefitting just a tad bit more from all that "smushing."

In most respects this is not a big deal. As we earlier noted, the human body is remarkably adept at drawing the oxygen it needs from its surroundings. But these small differences do add up over time, and one place some researchers believe this might be playing out is in the mental health of people who live at higher elevations. Multiple studies have revealed a strong correlation between altitude and the risk of depression and suicide—and those associations appear to hold strong even when researchers have adjusted for other factors known to impact mental health, like overall health, income, gun ownership, and religion.[18] What's more, scientists who have tracked people who move from lower elevations to higher elevations have found a striking connection to increased symptoms of depression, anxiety, and suicidal thoughts.[19] At the heart of these associations, many researchers believe, is the effect of hypobaric hypoxia, an imbalance of oxygen availability to tissue needs, on the metabolism of serotonin. This neurotransmitter has an outsize impact on cognition, memory, and especially mood, and its production is sensitive to oxygen availability.[20]

If the relatively small differences in pressure and oxygen saturation that exist between places like San Francisco and Denver can impact serotonin production and thus mental health outcomes, could even more oxygen, literally pressed into action by higher pressures, lead to better mental health outcomes? As of the mid-2010s, despite more than a century of history of hyperbaric exploration, there were virtually no credible studies on the clinical effectiveness of hyperbaric oxygen therapy for the treatment of mental health issues like anxiety and depression.[21]

Over the past decade that has begun to change—in no small part because Chinese researchers have taken the lead in investigating the connection between hyperbaric treatment and mental health. In 2013, researchers at Nanjing University of Medical Sciences in eastern China took 60 patients who had suffered from a brain injury and were experiencing the common symptom of convalescent depression and divided them into two groups, one that received 30 sessions of HbOT and the other that was treated with a commonly used short-term antidepressant. The results were profound. Depression among the drug-treated group was improved almost exactly in line with what prior studies suggested the drug should do. (In other words, it was nominally effective.) The HbOT-treated group not only experienced far more profound improvements in the rate and severity of convalescent depression, but they also experienced quicker recovery from the underlying brain injury.[22]

Two years later, another group of Chinese researchers, this time from Hangzhou Hospital in a southwest suburb of Shanghai, used a similar process for evaluating HbOT as a treatment for depression among patients after a stroke. Again, the investigation showed that hyperbaric therapy was more effective than drugs alone—and patients who received both drugs and multiple HbOT sessions fared even better.[23]

Then, in 2017, researchers from Zhengzhou University, about 400 miles south of Beijing, once again found that HbOT was an effective treatment for depression and anxiety—this time for a group of patients who were recovering from spinal cord injuries.[24]

All these studies were performed on patients who were suffering from depression that was connected to other diseases and injuries. And the results of each investigation might lead to a sort of chicken-and-egg question about whether the test subjects' improved mental health was helping with their recovery or whether their recovery was driving improvements in mental health.

We've come to believe it's both. And we are not alone. Writing in the journal *Medicine*, the authors of the study on the effects on HbOT on the mental health outcomes of people recovering from spinal cord injury suggested "there is a vicious cycle between psychological factors and functional impairment in spinal cord injury patients with psychological problems, and hyperbaric oxygen is able to break this vicious cycle." And if HbOT relieves depression, anxiety, and other negative emotions, the researchers continued, it may "strengthen patients' resolve to overcome disease; and let patients more actively participate in rehabilitation training, forming a virtuous circle."

Must you first be injured or debilitated with a disease, which then causes depressive symptoms, in order to derive a mental health benefit from hyperbaric oxygen? It might seem reasonable to say "of course not." It would seem to stand to reason that hyperbaric treatment would be effective no matter how a person's depression came to be. But, as of yet, there has been little academic research on whether generalized depression and other mental health conditions are alleviated by higher levels of pressurized oxygen.

From a research logistics perspective, the early focus on convalescent depression does make sense. People who are already hospitalized follow-ing a brain injury, stroke, or spinal cord injury constitute a test population with fewer confounding variables at play than in a nonhospitalized group of people who are suffering from depression.

Psychiatrists in Israel have taken at least one step in this direction. In the fall of 2021, they reported the results of a study that examined the potential benefits of greater oxygen saturation at normal atmospheric pressure. To conduct that study, the researchers divided about 50 peo-ple who were suffering from depression into two groups. The first group received enriched oxygen each night while they slept. The second group went through the same process but received a placebo dose of average, or-dinary air. The study was also double-blinded—the individuals who were administering the treatments and assessing the test subjects' symptoms were also unaware of who was getting the enriched air and who was get-ting the placebo.[25]

Placebos can be powerful. And indeed, about 25 percent of the in-dividuals in the normal oxygen group showed a decline in the severity of their symptoms over the course of the four-week treatment. That's in line with studies of antidepressant drugs, which have shown that 20 to 40 percent of people who take a pharmaceutical placebo will experience an improvement in their symptoms.

But among those who received the enriched air, about 70 percent ex-perienced improvements, including a decrease in suicidal thoughts, feel-ings of guilt, and insomnia. And that's better than the effects we typically expect of antidepressants, which result in improvements 40 to 60 percent of the time.[26]

Two things about this study jump out at us. First, it would appear that even *thinking* more consciously about our breathing—as study par-ticipants in both the test and control groups had to do each night as they settled down connected to a machine that gently pushed air through their nostrils—can be beneficial. Second, even small increases in oxygen at normal atmospheric pressure can be powerful—and without the side effects that can sometimes come with pharmaceutical interventions, including nausea, weight gain, fatigue, sleep problems, agitation, and decreased sex drives.

Even small increases in oxygen at normal atmospheric pressure can be powerful.

Elana experienced several of those symptoms when she was prescribed escitalopram, which is often sold under the brand names Cipralex and Lexapro.

"It felt magical at first," the 32-year-old forensic accountant from Washington, DC, recalled. "For a few months, it felt like I was literally breathing easier. I could get out of bed in the morning so much easier. There were side effects, but it felt like a fair trade for what I'd gained."

After a few years of using escitalopram, though, Elana began to wonder whether she really benefited from the tradeoff. "I was definitely happier and healthier in some really important ways, but my sex life was nonexistent," she said. "I have this amazing partner who has been supportive of me in so many ways, but I just had no desire or interest. This thing that had been an important part of our life together—even when I was depressed—went away."

Experiences like Elana's may be one of the major reasons that, in the long term, many people who take antidepressants end up reporting no overall improvement in their quality of life.[27] That's not everyone's experience. Some people who have been on these medications for many years have had lots of success, and few if any side effects, and would never even consider changing course. But even advocates for antidepressants, like research psychologist Gemma Lewis, recognize the vast limitations. "There's strong evidence that antidepressants can be effective for people experiencing a wide range of depressive symptoms," Lewis said in 2021. She conceded, however, that pharmaceuticals "do not work for everybody" with depression.[28]

Fortunately, the psychiatrist who had prescribed escitalopram to Elana didn't simply tell her to try another drug. "She listened to me and I felt like she was empathizing with what I was going through—this feeling that I'd taken one big step in the right direction but an equally big step the other way," Elana explained. "And she said, 'You know what? Let's try something else.'"

Over the next six weeks, Elana tapered her antidepressant use, reducing her dose at a rate prescribed by her doctor. At the same time she began making weekly visits to a Restore center in North Bethesda, Maryland, for one-hour mHbOT sessions.

"I was worried there would be a return to the symptoms that the drugs had helped alleviate but, at least for me, that never happened," she said. "I was still waking up better, happier, more ready to face the world. And the things I was missing from life—that really important part of our life together—started to return, and now it's like it was in the best times of being together. In fact, I think that now is the best time of our relationship."

We can think of no better outcome. And it's all likely due to something happening deep inside our cells.

Cellular Psychology

The biochemical mechanisms at the heart of life-changing stories like Elana's are likely to be the subject of a lot of scientific exploration for years to come. But one leading hypothesis among many researchers is that the administration of high levels of oxygen at pressures greater than one atmosphere results in an up to 20-fold increase in the proportion of dissolved oxygen in our blood.[29] What that means, in turn, is that the primary consumer of oxygen in the bloodstream, the mitochondria packed into nearly every cell in our bodies (red blood cells being the exception), are able to feast and feast—and increase their production of energy as a result.

Does it matter that hyperbaric therapy provides this benefit for only a short time? Yes, but in a surprising way. You may recall from our discussion of the varying levels of oxygen at different elevations that the human body is remarkably adept at getting used to whatever oxygen environment it finds itself in. As a result, when oxygen levels fall from the high levels that exist in hyperbaric treatments to the normal conditions that exist in the surrounding world, our bodies interpret the drop in O_2 as a hypoxic signal, even though there is, of course, no actual hypoxia occurring, activating a wide range of physiological responses that enhance cellular activity in a way that promotes wellness. This balance between states of increased and decreased oxygen has come to be known as the hyperoxic-hypoxic paradox,[30] and it wouldn't exist if the oxygen environment lasted all the time. Thus, the short-term nature of this treatment is vital to its efficacy.

In the way we've come to think of interventions like cryotherapy, heat immersion, and hyperbaric oxygen, that short-term production of energy is capacity that people can build on in other ways. For Elana, it appears to have been just what she needed to help her get out of bed in the morning and feel a little better about her life—without the drugs. That allowed her to mitigate a headwind—the side effects that came along with her daily dose of escitalopram. And that, in turn, helped her accentuate a tailwind, the connection and support she had from her partner. The virtuous cycle was activated.

The short-term nature of this treatment is vital to its efficacy.

What she did next is important: She invested some of the capacity into other interventions. After six months of visiting Restore for hyperbaric oxygen, she decided to try out cryotherapy, which added just a few minutes to each visit but turned out to be effective at reducing the long-term pain she had been carrying in her knees for more than a decade after she stopped playing soccer in college. That allowed her to do something she would never have considered when it was hard to just get out of bed. "I started going on a run around my neighborhood every morning," she said. "And the more I ran, the better I felt, and eventually I got to the place where even though I've still kept up the habit of going to Restore every week, I don't worry at all when I miss a week or even two. Other parts of my life help sustain me, keep me happy—and actually I have gotten used to feeling happier each day."

Unlike cold therapy and heat immersion, there aren't so many do-it-yourself ways to mimic the effects of hyperbaric oxygen, but that doesn't mean you can't benefit in similar ways through other means.

For one thing, as the team from Ben-Gurion University in Israel demonstrated, even "normobaric" oxygen—higher concentrations of O_2 provided at regular atmospheric pressure—can be beneficial. Others have found that this form of oxygen supplementation can be helpful for treating chronic decreases in the flow of blood into the brain,[31] and can mitigate neurological symptoms related to reduced outflow of blood from the brain, too.[32] These studies were performed under clinical conditions, but they were also conducted on people with severe illnesses. In contrast, commercial oxygen bars—of the sort that have popped up in the past decade in trendy towns all over the globe—are in no way a controlled clinical setting, but they also don't (and shouldn't) cater to people with debilitating illnesses, and they may be able to offer some of the benefits of the hyperoxic-hypoxic paradox to customers who purchase sessions that typically last for up to 20 minutes. The same might be true for over-the-counter oxygen canisters, which have become especially popular in recent years at high-elevation ski resorts and on the sidelines of sporting events (although there's little independent research that has been conducted on these interventions).

And there is, of course, another age-old way to get more oxygen into our bodies, and into the hungry "mouths" of the mitochondria in our cells: simple exercise. The combination of aerobic and resistance training has been shown to improve mitochondrial respiration in our cells,[33] in no small part because it increases the rate at which oxygen flows into and out of our lungs. This is so obvious, and yet so routinely ignored, that researchers from the University of Naples in Italy jocosely called it a "novel" tool to protect mitochondrial health[34] and one of their counterparts in Australia whimsically noted that such findings are "a breath of fresh air."[35]

Regarding fresh air, there's really no substitute. A lot of people think that toxins are the biggest problem of polluted air, and the fine particulate matter often found in urban and industrial communities is indeed a tremendous hazard. But a big part of the reason that we tend to feel so cruddy on days in which the air quality index rises from green to yellow or yellow to orange or onward from there to the devastatingly unhealthy "maroon" level (which is essentially equivalent to chain-smoking) isn't just the presence of toxic chemicals in our air, it's the absence of oxygen.[36] Thus, anything you can do to help ensure you're breathing in the freshest air possible—including using air filters and plants that help recycle air indoors[37] and recycling the air inside by opening windows when the air outside is healthiest—is a positive step toward this part of wellness.

Finally, it may also be helpful to engage in practices that center the act of breathing with intentionality. That might include meditations such as those made popular by the late Zen Master Thich Nhat Hanh, who encouraged his followers to engage in mantras such as "Breathing out, I feel at ease. Breathing in, I smile. Breathing out, I release. Breathing in, I dwell in the present moment." It might also include nasal-only or pursed-lip breathing, the latter of which can help you slow your breathing and bring in more air, and has been shown to make exercise easier, reduce stress, and even help combat some diseases.[38]

*Engage in practices that center the act
of breathing with intentionality.*

Inherent in intentional breathing exercises is a simple premise and a rather profound promise: We breathe in and out more than 20,000 times a day, and every one of those breaths is an opportunity to get just a little bit closer to a state of hyper wellness.

chapter 6

hydration

As Tilly approached her 50th birthday, she began experiencing a symptom of aging almost everyone encounters at some point in their life: back pain.

Tilly did what many people do; she went to a chiropractor. And the chiropractor did what many chiropractors do; she used pressure to make small adjustments that realigned Tilly's joints to decrease pain and increase her range of motion. The doctor also gave Tilly some exercises intended to help maintain those adjustments.

But then the chiropractor told Tilly something she had never considered before: One of the most important ways to alleviate back pain is the seemingly simple act of staying adequately hydrated.

Much of this has to do with the makeup and purpose of our intervertebral discs, the small "cushions" that act as shock absorbers along our spines. The inner part of each of these discs is made up of a soft inner circle called the nucleus pulposus, and a tougher outer structure composed of layers of tissue called the annulus fibrosus, and both parts rely on hydration to remain "marshmallow-like" in their consistency. When intervertebral discs are insufficiently hydrated, they shrink, resulting in insufficient support for the spine, which often leads to stress, swelling, slipped discs, and pinched nerves, among other sources of pain.

Hypohydration—a lack of adequate water in the body—has also been shown to decrease cognitive function, increase fatigue, promote negative moods, and accentuate the perception of pain,[1] all of which can make it even harder to tolerate the symptoms of underhydrated intervertebral discs. What's more, intervertebral tissue often degenerates with aging,[2] making it harder to stay ahead of the hydration curve to keep back problems at bay.

And that is why Tilly's chiropractor referred her to a Restore center near her home in Texas for an IV drip, a practice that Tilly has now made a regular part of her life.

"I feel the benefits right away," she said. "And when I leave Restore after a drip I feel invigorated. I feel I have way more energy and it just makes my day."

By now, you'll recognize Tilly's experience with IV fluids as a right-away benefit that created capacity for other steps on the virtuous cycle leading toward hyper wellness. Part of this immediate feeling of improved wellness is likely a result of the nutrients in her drip (a subject we'll dive into in chapter 9). But a big part of her right-away response to this form of therapy is simply that the tissues in her body, and especially those that support her back, are being supported with additional hydration.

"I feel I have way more energy and it just makes my day."

After oxygen, there's nothing our bodies need more than water. Even the hardest tissues in our bodies, our bones, are about 20 percent water. Our muscles and brains are about 75 percent water. Our blood is about 85 percent. But these figures vary as a factor of wellness and aging. The total water content of the biologically youngest, most hyper well adults in the world is closer to 70 percent; the biologically oldest and chronically ill are often closer to 40 percent.[3]

These are not spurious relationships. In addition to the roles we noted earlier, water also supports the regulation of temperature, the function of organs, the transport of nutrients, the movement of oxygen, the lubrication of joints, and the removal of waste from our bodies.

Despite the commonsensical nature of the role of hydration—and the ease at which most of us can put water into our bodies at virtually any time—dehydration is rampant.

While it's commonly reported that 75 percent of Americans are chronically dehydrated, that figure appears to be an exceedingly inexact extrapolation of several studies and surveys. In truth, we don't know, because each person's water needs vary as a condition of their body size, work conditions, exercise habits, food choices, and age. It also turns out to be a hard thing to quantify, even among people of similar age and body types, because water is stored in our bodies inside each cell, in the space between cells, in blood plasma, in the gastrointestinal tract, and in the bladder. So, while terms like "dehydration" and "hyperhydration" commonly refer to the water content of a person's whole body, in truth these conditions can simultaneously and independently exist in different areas of the body.[4] It's possible to be dehydrated in one place and hyperhydrated in another at the same time!

That doesn't mean that we're clueless about people's general state of hydration. We do know, for instance, that about 7 percent of American adults don't drink water at all. (These people are getting water in other ways, of course, because if they weren't then they would be dead, but they certainly aren't getting hydration in what is generally the most immediately available and efficient manner.) In the same survey from which that estimate was derived, just about 1 in 4 Americans reported drinking eight cups of water or more, which has long been the standard advice many doctors give on water consumption, and thus that survey might be the genesis for the 75 percent stat that shows up in the media so often.[5]

We do know that *actual* chronic dehydration—a state in which a person is consistently losing more water than they are taking in over a long period of time, leading to organ malfunction and aggravating states of disease—is particularly common among older adults,[6] but the truth is that there are few people who haven't screwed up this fundamental part of life at least a few times, and many people have experienced the symptoms of profound dehydration multiple times.

Even exceptional athletes are at risk. After Minnesota Vikings tackle Korey Stringer collapsed on a practice field in July 2001 and died early the next morning, many critics noted that the tragedy was preventable: If Stringer had been properly hydrated, it's almost certain that he would still be here today. And yet, two decades later, troublingly similar incidents are still occurring, perhaps most notably the death of University of Maryland offensive lineman Jordan McNair, who collapsed during a practice in May 2018 and died two weeks later, and whose death has also been attributed to heat stroke caused in part by dehydration.

If athletes who are surrounded at nearly all times by the best athletic trainers in the world are still at risk of getting hydration wrong, it might seem like this is a tremendously complicated part of our lives. It's not. There is, however, far more at play than "drink plenty of water," which is the hydration advice most people get—if they get any advice on hydration whatsoever.

But it's also true that of all the elements of hyper wellness, this may be the *easiest* place from which to get a foothold on the feel-better-do-more cycle—and something of a secret weapon against some of the most common and debilitating health challenges in our modern world.

Heads Up

Chronic migraine is one of the most common neurologic disorders around the world.[7] Many people spend years, decades, or even their entire lives seeking a cure, going from specialist to specialist, trying drug after drug, without meaningful alleviation of this horrible experience.

Migraine is a complex disorder, and there's no one-size-fits-all solution. Studies have revealed mutations in several genes that can indicate a propensity for migraines and can be passed down through generations, and given that women suffer from migraines at a rate three times greater than men, it's likely that hormonal or X-chromosome-linked factors are at play.[8]

Given these complexities, it might seem crazy to suggest a simple trip to the water faucet could be life-changing for many people. But the results of studies examining the impact of basic hydration on migraines reveal a rather shocking truth: Many people who suffer from headaches so bad that they seek a doctor's care could significantly and sometimes entirely alleviate their suffering with water alone!

That was the case for many of the 256 women who checked into headache clinics at two hospitals in Tehran, Iran, in the late 2010s, and who were enrolled in a simple study in which their headache, frequency, and duration were assessed for 30 days thereafter. Among the other things researchers watched for was how much and how often the patients drank water. Those who drank more water had fewer headaches, less painful headaches, and shorter headaches.[9] That wasn't an outlying result: Researchers from other parts of the world have found dehydration can cause horrible headaches on its own and also exacerbate migraines that stem from other underlying medical conditions.[10] Thus, for many people, water is as effective as powerful drugs.

Here's one of the main reasons why: Using what was then a relatively new technology, magnetic resonance imaging–based computerized brain volumetry, German researchers found in the early 2000s that less than a day of inadequate water intake could significantly change the volume of a person's brain.[11] When a lack of hydration leads to shrinkage, the brain pulls away from the skull, putting pressure on the cranial nerves, which, when stimulated in this way, can trigger inflammation in the cerebral blood vessels and meninges, the layers of tissue that envelop the brain. It takes only a 1 percent difference in brain size to result in symptoms like throbbing headaches, sensitivity to light and sound, and nausea.

For many people, water is as effective as powerful drugs.

If you're not someone who has suffered from chronic debilitating headaches, it might be tempting to blame the victims here, but we'd suggest holding your fire. As we'll explain shortly, it's not just migraines that are sometimes caused by a lack of thoughtfulness about hydration.

If you have battled migraines, it might be tempting to dismiss a discussion about this research as condescending. Before you do that, consider this: How many doctors have spent more than a few seconds speaking to you about proper hydration?

"My doctors definitely didn't do that," said Lauren, a physics instructor in her early 40s who lives and teaches on the Kansas side of the Kansas City border, "and when I think back on all the conversations I've had, I wonder if they all just figured that it was so obvious that it went without saying. I felt stupid about it for a long time."

It wasn't stupid, though. Because the truth is that doctors don't often talk to their patients about hydration, and quizzes of medical professionals on basic matters of hydration have revealed huge deficits in knowledge about this fundamental part of wellness. Physicians often even acknowledge that they don't get enough water themselves. In one survey, about a third of the doctors who filled out a questionnaire about hydration said they didn't have access to easily available drinking water at work; of those who did, a third said they don't bother to make use of it. Nearly half rated their own personal hydration habits as "bad" and only 2 percent said their hydration status was "excellent."[12]

It's no wonder Lauren didn't understand hydration might be the key to alleviating her suffering: Her doctors either didn't know themselves or didn't prioritize this aspect of wellness over other interventions.

Lauren had been fighting migraines since she was in her mid-20s. At first, she attributed the headaches to the stress of graduate school. She also recognized this had been a period of her life when she was drinking a lot of coffee, and under the advice of her doctor, she had temporarily cut back to just one cup a day. But it turned out that, as for many people, the caffeine in a cup of coffee could help alleviate the symptoms of her migraines, so her doctor suggested she move on to other interventions.[13]

"It feels like I tried a hundred different things over the years," she said. "There were over-the-counter drugs and prescription drugs. Some worked a little bit and some didn't work at all. The ones that did work all had side effects I didn't like."

It wasn't migraines that first got Lauren interested in IV drip therapy. Instead, it was travel. In February 2022, the day before a trip to Cancun for a friend's wedding, Lauren and three other bridesmaids visited a Restore center in Overland Park, Kansas, for a pre-travel IV session, a common practice among people who are hoping to boost their body's natural defenses before getting on a plane.

"I almost didn't go for the IV because I was having some initial migraine aura," she said, referencing the symptoms some people get preceding a migraine headache. "I decided to try to push through, though, and we all went together, and it was just a really relaxing experience."

That night, as she got ready for bed, Lauren realized the migraine she feared was on its way hadn't materialized. "It really hit me, right there. There had been a few times over the years when my migraine had gotten so bad that I went to the hospital, and I got an IV drip as part of my treatment. And I just realized that maybe I didn't have to wait for a migraine to get bad before that could be helpful," she said.

In a paper published in 2012, University of California San Francisco neurologists Amy Gelfand and Peter Goadsby noted that while many studies of migraine therapies included IV fluids as part of the treatment protocol alongside medications or other therapeutic interventions, it has been rare for researchers to evaluate how much the IV alone might contribute to migraine improvement. "But," the researchers wrote, "fluid replacement is arguably an underappreciated aspect of acute migraine therapy."[14]

Encouraged by that first experience with the IV drip, Lauren began focusing on staying better hydrated all the time—carrying around a one-liter water bottle she seeks to finish by lunchtime, then refill, and finish again by dinner. She also began trying to get a drip whenever she was experiencing migraine aura. That proved difficult, so instead she began to make a weekly proactive visit to a studio near her home. "That turned out to be the combination that has worked for me," she said. "I've gone from seven or eight bad migraines a month to one or two, and there have been a few months that I didn't have a single one. It's been life-changing."

Life-changing! That's a term we keep hearing again and again. And it absolutely fills our hearts.

"I've gone from seven or eight bad migraines a month to one or two, and there have been a few months that I didn't have a single one. It's been life-changing."

I Heart Water

For more than a year after he was diagnosed with atrial fibrillation, Jude dutifully documented his triggers—the sorts of situations that most often resulted in an episode of "runaway" heart palpitations.

"My doctor was honest with me and told me that the best thing I could possibly do would be to drop a lot of weight. That could make a big difference, but it also wasn't something I could do quickly," he said. "For a quicker impact, there were drugs and procedures, but I wanted to avoid all that for as long as I could, if possible."

Jude figured that if he could determine what his most common triggers were—and work hard to avoid those things in his life—he could buy himself some time for other healthy actions to have an effect.

It was obvious from the onset that after a night of poor sleep, his heart would often get away from him, so he worked hard to create a cool, comfortable, dark environment, set a constant bedtime, and steadfastly followed a "no computer screens" rule in his bedroom.

Getting a good night of sleep created a bit of a tailwind for the next major trigger he recognized: caffeine. When it comes to hydration, the world's most popular stimulant impacts different people in different ways. Sometimes it can help—as it did for Lauren and her migraines. Other times it can be problematic—and that was the case for Jude, as it is for many people with AFib.

As a lifetime coffee drinker, the literature professor had long relied on a couple cups in the morning to "get going," and another to "keep going" after lunch. "On a university campus, coffee is so ingrained into the culture that it's hard to get away from," he said. "There are days that I'd have six cups without even thinking about it." Over time Jude noticed that on the days on which he could skip some or most of those shots—either by avoiding it altogether or drinking decaf—he was less likely to have an AFib episode, and since he wasn't feeling nearly as tired anymore, anyway, he was able to cut back on that, too.

The last trigger, though, was the hardest to accept. Jude knew that exercise would be essential to getting rid of the weight he needed to lose to put his condition into remission, but his exercise sessions were often cut short—or shortly followed by—an uncontrollably pounding heartbeat.

"That was demoralizing," he said. "It was like a double-edged sword. Exercise was the path to naturally limiting my episodes, but it was also causing my episodes."

His doctor told him that while quick bursts of exercise are often associated with triggering AFib, a slower progression into each exercise session—stretching, then light weight training, then light cardio, then a gradually more intense workout—works to keep a lot of patients from having an episode. But Jude also learned that AFib events are much more likely to happen when exercise happens without adequate hydration,[15] chiefly because dehydration impacts the balance of electrolytes, the minerals in our bodies that carry an electric charge—and AFib, at its core, happens as a result of disorganized electrical signals.[16]

The solution was simple. For starters, Jude replaced his entire coffee habit with a water habit. "Instead of waking up and drinking two cups of coffee, I wake up and drink two cups of water," he said. "And instead of having a cup of coffee after lunch, I fill up a bottle of water and work on that for the rest of the day."

Jude also began making biweekly visits to a Restore center a few miles south of his home in Berkeley, California, where his "signature shot" includes an IV drip with magnesium. He also started to take a daily potassium supplement.

That wasn't a shot in the dark. In a cohort study of more than 2,500 emergency-room admissions of patients with atrial fibrillation, researchers from Austria's Medical University of Vienna found that the intravenous administration of those two electrolytes increased the rates of "spontaneous conversion," a natural return to normal heart rhythm without the need for the quick, low-energy shocks that doctors use to restore a patient to regular heart rhythm. "This approach might lessen the need for pharmacologic intervention and potential adverse effects," the researchers wrote.[17]

Jude feels the evidence for that is strong in his specific situation.

"I made a lot of changes in a short amount of time," he said, "so it's hard to say whether these decisions worked separately or together, but I know that keeping my hydration good and my electrolytes balanced has been huge for preventing more episodes. I still usually do a slow warmup when I'm exercising, but I can absolutely go from zero to a full sprint without worrying about triggering my AFib."

What that has meant for Jude is a two-workouts-per-day habit that resulted in significant weight loss following his initial diagnosis. "I'm not on any drugs and I haven't had to have any procedures," he said. "I know that the cellular damage in my heart is still there, so I'm not cured, so to speak, but I never drop out of normal rhythm anymore. It just doesn't happen, and I credit my hydration routine for that change."

All this raises an important question: What if we didn't wait until people were in dire straits to supplement their hydration and electrolyte balance?

What if we didn't wait until people were in dire straits?

The Well-Hydrated Lifestyle

Even though water makes up the vast majority of most human bodies, impacts metabolism, maintains electrolyte balance, and plays numerous other functions related to human wellness—and even though we've known all this for a long time—there has been little research about what happens to our brains when water becomes scarcer in our bodies.

Jianfen Zhang and Na Zhang are on a mission to change that. Technically, the two Peking University researchers work for a laboratory dedicated to understanding the impact of food on human health. But in the mid 2010s, when they first teamed up to investigate the effects of hydration on the cognitive performance of young adults, they realized something striking. While the foods we eat can have a substantial impact on our cognitive health, the amount of water we drink has an even greater impact.[18] From that point on, the two Zhangs have been insatiable in their efforts to understand the specific ways in which hydration impacts our brains, completing several studies each year demonstrating that dehydration impairs episodic memory and mood,[19] along with brain imaging research that shows that even a short-term decrease in water consumption can impact the density of gray matter (which controls movement, memory, and emotions) and white matter (which conducts, processes, and sends signals) in the brain.[20]

The fascinating thing about these researchers' work is that it has mostly been conducted on relatively young people in average health, thus demonstrating that you don't have to have an underlying medical condition like back pain, migraines, or AFib to accentuate the hydration tailwind.

That was the case for Tomomi, a physical trainer in Sacramento, California, who returned to school in her mid 30s in hopes of developing the skills she would need to open her own business. "I'd always done well in school before, and I was ready to crush it in my MBA program," she said. "But I found that my brain got tired of reading and writing and thinking so much faster than when I was in college the first time."

In August 2022, Tomomi tried an IV infusion for the first time. And something changed.

"I'm a big believer in 'mind over matter,' so I'm willing to accept that it could have all been in my head, but after my drip I walked out of there feeling so good," Tomomi said. "If I'm being honest, I don't care as long as it's safe. It's hard to explain adequately, but my brain felt younger and more eager to learn." She now does an IV drip at least once every few weeks, "and it has the same effect on me as the very first one did."

The big takeaway from Tomomi's story is that there wasn't anything "wrong" with her. She wasn't suffering from a disease. She was simply experiencing the impacts of aging on her cognitive health. And this is one of the big differences between the hyper wellness lifestyle and traditional medicine. The virtuous cycle doesn't need to begin with pain or disease. It can start long before the sorts of things that trigger a visit to the doctor—and in our view it's so much better if it does.

On H$_2$O and IVs

If dehydration is the cause—or at least an aggravating factor—for conditions like chronic back pain, migraine, and atrial fibrillation, wouldn't a better, easier, and cheaper solution simply be drinking more water? If cognitive performance can be improved with a few more glasses of water each day, isn't that where we should all begin?

First and foremost, yes. But there's more to it than that. For one thing, everyone's water needs are different, and the standard admonition to "drink at least eight 8-ounce glasses of water a day" (which many health promotion organizations have reduced to "drink 8×8") does not appear to be backed by any sort of scientific evidence. When Heinz Valtin, a highly regarded physiologist who taught at Dartmouth College, went looking for the origins of this common advice in the early 2000s, the best he could surmise was that it started back in the 1970s as part of a brief section on hydration at the end of a book called *Nutrition for Good Health*, in which the authors wrote—without any reference—that "somewhere around 6 to 8 glasses per 24 hours" was a good target. At best, this was "shoot from the hip" health advice, accentuated in no small part by the fact that the authors also suggested that soft drinks and beer were suitable substitutes for water![21]

Valtin's now-infamous diatribe on "drink 8×8" was apoplectic in tone. "As we look around us in our daily activities, we can observe how slavishly the exhortation is being followed. Everywhere, people are carrying bottles of water and taking frequent sips from them," he wrote. "For some the bottle has even become a security blanket."[22]

Valtin was being histrionic. There's no reason to denigrate people who habitually carry water. But there's such a thing as too much of a good thing. Our kidneys can remove only about one gallon of water every four hours, but unless you're engaged in vigorous exercise, it's unlikely you need to be running your kidneys at max capacity, and overhydration can lead to a dangerous imbalance of the electrolytes our bodies need to carry signals from cell to cell, a condition sometimes called "water intoxication" that can cause disorientation, nausea, and vomiting, and which in some cases can lead to brain swelling.

Some have taken Valtin's screed, and observations about the rare dangers of water intoxication, to infer that people don't need to drink more water. That's not true. Most do! But the real point seems to be that everyone's needs are different—and data should prevail over slogans. A 5-foot-1 woman in her 20s who works as a roofer in Arizona is going to have different hydration needs than a 6-foot-4 man in his 40s who sits at a desk all day—and both of them will be much different from a 5-foot-7 woman in her 70s who plays tennis in the morning and swims in the afternoons.

Data should prevail over slogans.

What is by far most important, from our perspective, is whether someone's level of hydration equates to a greater state of wellness. And the best way to assess that is by first understanding your baseline. How much water are you already drinking each day? That's simple enough to quantify by keeping a journal. Things get a little more complicated when we recognize that a lot of our hydration doesn't come from water, but from other drinks. What's more, about 20 percent of our total hydrating intake comes from the foods we eat. Fortunately, there are several good smartphone apps that can help you quantify your normal "hydration budget."

When you go through this process, you're likely to recognize that you're not hydrating enough. It's important to remember, though, that whatever water you're taking in, from whatever source, is a tailwind that can be easily accentuated. Unless a physician tells you otherwise—and that's exceedingly unlikely—adding a single cup of water a day in the morning and another cup of water each afternoon is a good initial goal. Do that and track the results for a few weeks, then try to add either another daily cup of water at a time or an extra helping of a water-saturated food (cantaloupes, strawberries, watermelons, lettuce, cabbage, celery, spinach, and cooked squash are among the best, and yogurt, apples, grapes, oranges, carrots, cooked broccoli, pears, pineapple, bananas, avocados, and corn are up there, too).[23] Improve and assess. Improve a little more and assess again.

Does the equivalent of six servings of water each day lead to a life of less pain, more mobility, clearer thoughts, and more energy, while seven glasses lead to all that but also more trips to the restroom? Well then, six it should be.

Are the equivalent of ten or twelve servings of water still not sufficient to make a dent in many of the conditions that water is expected to be helpful for, including headaches, joint pain, sleep quality, and clarity of thought? Perhaps then the problem isn't a lack of water but an excess of aging—which, as we earlier noted, makes it harder for the body to hold on to the water it brings in. (It's important to remember that aging doesn't mean "old age" but is rather a concept that should be considered to be proportionally inverse to wellness. We are all experiencing biological aging from the moment of our births!) That's when it becomes worthwhile to explore regular supplementation of hydration and other nutrients, perhaps via an IV, as we will discuss further in chapter 9. But, again, this is a decision that should be driven by personal data—not generalized advice or platitudes.

The bottom line is this: Hydration is an undervalued and often overlooked part of holistic wellness. And since it's perhaps the most easily changeable of all the elements of hyper wellness, it can be a great place to start your journey on the virtuous cycle.

chapter 7

rest

For a long time, Becca was jealous of her husband, Rob, who always seemed to be able to fall asleep the moment his head hit the pillow.

"At the end of the day, we'd kiss each other and say goodnight, and he'd lie down and be snoring almost immediately," the pediatric nurse from New Orleans recalled. "And I'd lie there and stare at the ceiling and think, 'I'm losing out on the sleep I need. What is it that he is doing right that I'm doing wrong? Why is he such a good sleeper?'"

Sometimes, Becca said, that would be the bitter last thought she would have before she would finally drift off—and she would stew over it the next day at work as she tried to stay alert and focused on her important job.

Becca isn't alone in her jealousy of people, like her husband, who seem to sleep so well. A survey conducted in 2022 by Gallup found that only about a third of Americans would rate their sleep as "high-quality."[1] Perhaps not coincidentally, about two-thirds of people say they want more sleep more than they want better sex![2] It's possible this says as much about the quality of our sex lives as it does about the quality of our sleeping lives, but statistics like these are complicated in other ways, too—and most of all by the fact that many people don't know what actually constitutes good sleep. As such, the status of our collective slumber might be, and in fact probably is, even more dire than the surveys suggest.

That became clear to Becca not long after Rob was diagnosed with obstructive sleep apnea, a common affliction in which a person's airway periodically collapses, causing them to stop breathing and disturbing their sleep. It turned out Rob wasn't falling asleep so quickly because he was a "good sleeper." He was falling asleep so quickly because the "mini wake-ups" he was experiencing each night were preventing him from getting restful slumber.

In reality, research suggests, the transition from wakefulness to sleep should be gradual, not immediate. As neurologist and sleep expert Chris Winter has noted, the idea that good sleep comes immediately when you lie down is one of many misconceptions that a lot of people have about this part of their lives. "It actually means he's sleep deprived," Winter said in 2021. "Like, his brain is so driven to find sleep that as soon as he gets into a relatively comfortable position, he's falling asleep."[3]

Winter's excellent book on healthy slumber, *The Sleep Solution*, was published in 2017, about a year before Rob's diagnosis. Becca said she and her husband both read it cover to cover, along with another book that came out that year, *Why We Sleep* by Matthew Walker.

"What I learned from this experience—what we both learned, actually—is that the way we thought about sleep was really skewed," Becca said. "We both used to think that sleep came down to minutes and hours. Like, how many minutes do you lie in bed before you fall asleep? The less the better, right? How many hours do you get each night, you know? The more the better. That's what we thought."

This is how many people quantify their sleep. Indeed, this is how many doctors tell people to quantify their sleep. That does make some sense, because most people can roughly estimate how many hours they get each night, but there are several problems with this. First off, and perhaps not surprisingly, these self-reported estimates are often wildly inaccurate.[4] Moreover, it takes an important and complex process that happens when we are unconscious and reduces it to a number. Worst of all, these numbers aren't even the most important piece of easily observable data. Indeed, when we consider the ways in which sleep serves as a tailwind or a headwind of wellness, it's clear that the most important thing to observe isn't how long it took us to fall asleep or how long we slept. It's how rested we feel.

"That seems so obvious to me now," Becca said. "But I'm in my 50s, and I've had some health problems before, so I've seen a lot of doctors in my lifetime. And sometimes I would be asked about how much I sleep, but never—like, absolutely never—about whether my sleep is actually restful."

Like many people with sleep apnea, Rob began using a continuous positive airway pressure (CPAP) machine, which uses constant air flow to keep his upper airway passages open, preventing the interruptions of breathing that result in sleep apnea.

"The funny thing to me is that with the breathing mask and all that tubing, he wasn't falling asleep as quickly, and I think the noise it made, which is sort of white noise, like just a soft hiss, was soothing to me. I'm pretty sure it helped me fall asleep easier," Becca said. "But that didn't help me feel better in the morning. So, all that time I was obsessing over the fact that I wasn't someone who falls asleep quickly—and it turns out that wasn't the problem."

Guided by the books by Winter and Walker, Becca became dedicated to "sleep regularity," getting to bed each night—and even on the weekends—by 10:30 p.m. and getting up each morning no later than 6 a.m. She also committed to "screenless evenings," shutting off her blue light–emitting television and computer screens by 8 p.m. each night, and slowly dimming the lights as bedtime approached. She set the bedroom thermostat to 65 degrees Fahrenheit—a few degrees cooler than she and

Rob kept the rest of their home. Finally, she sought to retrain her brain to associate her bed with sleep by not staying in bed whenever she struggled to fall asleep; instead she would get up, go to the living room, and work on a crossword puzzle under dim light until she was feeling sleepy again.

"I still have trouble falling asleep sometimes, but now I'm not obsessed," she said, "because what matters to me is whether I wake up feeling rested. When that happens, I know it, I feel it, my entire day is better because of it, and I can do so much more during the day!"

"What matters to me is whether I wake up feeling rested. When that happens, I know it, I feel it, my entire day is better because of it."

We think it's no coincidence that restful and restorative sleep offers a palpable, right-away perception of better wellness. Thus, like the other elements of wellness we've discussed so far, this is an aspect of our lives that offers us the capacity to take even more steps toward hyper wellness. But just as Becca first needed to change her perception of what constitutes good sleep, it's vital that we all develop a better understanding of what restfulness is, where it comes from, and how to accentuate the natural cycles that make it a force multiplier for accentuating wellness.

What Sleep Is... Really

Most people think of sleep as something that happens from the time they lose consciousness to the point they awaken, a period that generally occurs from late in the evening to sometime around sunrise. It's often commonly believed that sleep is an experience that gets deeper as the night goes on and becomes more shallow as the morning arrives, and if we were to track that on a chart, it might look something like this:

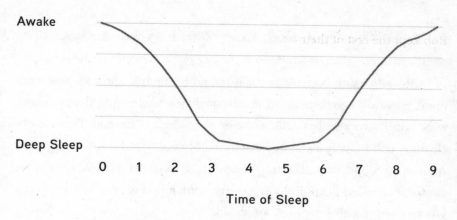

In this way of thinking about slumber, "good sleep" might be considered to be a period of unconsciousness that gets deeper quicker, and stays deeper longer. That experience might look like this:

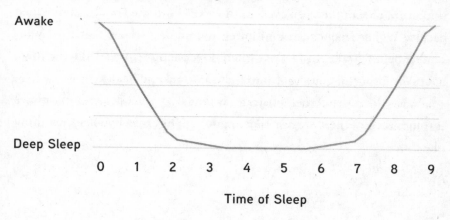

Historian Roger Ekirch is among those who have pointed out that this way of sleeping might not align with the way our ancestors slept.[5] Combing through thousands of years of literature, civic records, medical texts, and personal diaries from around the world, he has unearthed a compelling body of evidence suggesting that people experienced a "first sleep" of several hours, followed by a waking period that often lasted an hour or longer, followed by more sleep. That model fits nicely with what sleep actually is—a roller-coaster of variations in the electrical signals in our brains that lead to several distinct periods associated with dreaming, learning, emotional processing, and brain recovery, and characterized by rapid eye movement, or REM.

Understanding how we get to REM is important. The awake human brain generally operates at a high frequency and low amplitude. That's what our brainwaves look like when we're in the first stage of the sleep cycle, in which we've gone to bed but have not yet entered unconsciousness. As we enter light sleep, the frequency falls and the amplitude rises. This continues as we descend into deep sleep, which is characterized by a very low frequency and very high amplitude of electrical signals, and during which our brain releases neurotransmitters that signal our cells to enter into a period of repair.

But this isn't when REM happens. In fact, we don't get to that vitally important part of the sleep cycle until we've "bottomed out" and returned back to higher frequencies and lower amplitudes—those that closely resemble being awake. In fact, we often do leave our slumber during these hours for a short amount of time. That's normal and healthy.

What the research demonstrates is that sleep includes multiple cycles through each of these stages. Thus, a good night of sleep looks something like this:

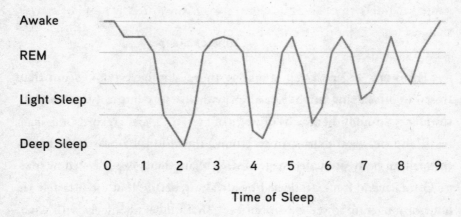

learning, emotional processing, and brain recovery, and characterized by

Good sleep comes as we move from wakefulness to light sleep to deep sleep, back up into light sleep, and then into REM. And if we briefly come out of sleep during REM, that's OK. Because the brain patterns between these stages of sleep are similar, this sort of shift comes as the result of a smooth transition of electrical activity in our brains.

What we don't want to see are sudden shifts—brain patterns, for instance, that indicate a jump from deep sleep to REM or, even worse, full wakefulness. But that's what a lot of people experience every night of their lives.

That was the case for Becca's husband, Rob, whose apnea was jarring him out of deep sleep multiple times each night, preventing the smooth and healthy transitions that provide the full benefits of each stage of sleep.

"I'd get out of bed and it was like I hadn't slept at all," he said. "I was so tired all the time, and I just thought that's what life was supposed to feel like, because I couldn't really remember a time when it hadn't been that way."

For Rob, sleep had become a powerful headwind to wellness—and owing to the mask and tangle of tubes, not even the CPAP machine was helping.

"I was too tired to exercise, so I'd been gaining weight, and it didn't help matters that because I felt exhausted all the time I didn't feel like I had the energy to cook anything healthy, so on the nights it was my turn to cook I always managed to convince Becca to let me take her out or have something delivered, and our choices were rarely healthy, and of course that just leads to more weight, which makes it even harder to exercise, and I felt trapped."

Rob knew he needed to find a way out of this paradox. And when a friend told him that he had been sleeping better after using the sauna at the local gym, Rob figured he'd give it a try.

There's no way to know for certain whether the sauna was helping Rob move more gently from one stage of sleep to another. (While Rob now uses an Oura Ring to track his sleep, he didn't back then.) But the difference he felt each morning when he woke up was profound.

"When I say the change was night and day, I don't just mean that in a metaphorical way," he said. "Before it had always felt like I was sort of sleep-walking through life. As soon as I started using the sauna, it was like there was this clarity to the difference between my nights and days. Now I know that's just what it feels like to actually be well rested."

That experience isn't unusual. In one study from researchers in Australia, sauna bathers reported no aspect of life was more powerfully affected by heat exposure than sleep. A stunning 84 percent of the study's participants reported improved sleep after sauna use.[6] Other research suggests that this effect might be connected to the ways in which sauna mimics the impacts of exercise in the human body, particularly by increasing the rate at which the body's temperature falls during sleep onset.[7] If the body's temperature is slightly raised before bedtime, as a result of either exercise or sauna, that fall will be more precipitous, triggering a more stable fluctuation across the various stages of sleep. But heat exposure has the advantage of not also triggering the release of endorphins, as exercise does, which is counterproductive to the onset of sleep for many people—which is why many sleep experts advise avoiding exercise, and especially vigorous exercise, right before bedtime.[8]

"Now I know that's just what it feels like to actually be well rested."

None of that is to suggest that heat exposure is the same thing as exercise from the standpoint of holistic wellness. It's not. Anyone who wishes to move toward hyper wellness needs both these elements in their life. Rob understood this, which is why he invested the capacity he was gaining from better sleep into more exercise—committing to starting every day with a workout and ending each day in a sauna.

"When you get up and you actually feel awake, it's a whole lot easier to start the day with a jog or a swim or some weightlifting, which is what I started doing each morning," he explained. "Within a few months, my weight was starting to drop, and that was helping me exercise even more."

In just a few months' time, he'd turned a powerful headwind into a tailwind.

And since weight loss is one of the most powerful ways to mitigate obstructive apnea,[9] Rob soon found that he was sleeping even better—so much so that, with the blessing of his doctor, he eventually ditched his CPAP machine.

That's something he wouldn't have dared to do if he hadn't been tracking his sleep, but after about a year of watching his sleep patterns gradually move from the interrupted patterns common to people with sleep apnea to the sine wave–like pattern that indicates a peaceful flow through each stage of sleep, he knew he was ready.

"I'm not quite to the point yet where I've completely forgotten what it was like when I was living in a constant state of exhaustion," he said, "but I haven't felt that way in a long time and, more and more these days, it feels like it was just a bad dream."

Tracking Sleep

While physical activity trackers are still far more common, there's probably no piece of modern heath tech that is more informative than the wide variety of sleep trackers that have become available in recent years. That's because while it's hard to perfectly quantify exercise without a tracker, it's easy enough to make a rough estimate of whether you got it and how vigorous it was. In contrast, while we can collect some important information about sleep quality when we wake up in the morning by assessing whether we feel well rested, most of what happened in the preceding hours is inaccessible to our conscious minds. It's impossible to know how many times you reached deep sleep, how many times you got to REM, and how smooth those transitions were.

That's where trackers come in. Some are designed to be worn as rings, others as bracelets, and others as patches. Most are measuring heart rate variability, which is a measurement of the variations in time between heartbeats, a good proxy for the brainwave activity that indicates different stages of sleep. Increasingly, some sleep trackers don't need to be worn at all—they clip onto your pillow or simply sit next to your bed, listening to the patterns of your breathing as an indicator of the electrical patterns in your brain.

What matters most is the data these devices provide, which shouldn't just provide a binary indication of "good" or "bad" sleep but should, at an absolute minimum, include consistently collected measurements of sleep duration, quality measured in a range, and time in phases.

We love it when we learn that first-timers at Restore are already tracking their sleep in this way, because it's one of the easiest ways to see that the immediate "feel better" experience they have when they step out of a cryotherapy spa, finish up mHbOT, or use an infrared sauna isn't just a short-term experience—it stokes a longer-term benefit and puts them onto the virtuous cycle.

Payton is a great example. The New Hampshire native was admittedly "obsessive" about his health and was already tracking activity, sleep, and general perceptions of wellness in a daily health journal he'd been keeping for nearly four years. "But I was always looking for ways to take the next step," he said.

He heard about cryotherapy in a podcast he was listening to while traveling for work. A few weeks later, he heard about it again on another show. And a couple days after that he heard about it yet again, on yet another show.

"I learned two things," Payton said. "One is that I definitely wanted to try cryo. The other is that maybe I needed to diversify the kinds of podcasts I'm listening to."

We wish we could take credit for the explosion of cryo conversations happening on hundreds of podcasts over the past few years. The truth is, though, that all this attention happened organically. Just as the story of Restore's founding began with a conversation between friends, many of the people who were responsible for the wave of podcasts focused on cryo had learned about this wellness modality from people close to them.

The good news about this sort of organic excitement is that people recognize it for what it is—the sort of authentic enthusiasm so rare in today's oversaturated world of slick advertising campaigns and paid influencers. But from the standpoint of a company trying to root itself in cold, hard science, the less good news is that while federal regulators control what companies can say about the health benefits of a modality like cryo, they can't control what is said by private citizens, like podcasters and other folks who share their own experiences on the internet.

We say "less good" rather than "bad" news because this is a double-edged sword. On the one hand, as we noted in the chapter dedicated to cold therapy, there's a lot of compelling, anecdotal evidence that suggests cryo has health benefits beyond what researchers have even attempted to investigate with double-blind, placebo-controlled studies (which are considered the "gold standard" for health research), and it's important for people to know what others are experiencing so they can best understand their own experiences. But on the other hand, Restore staff members often have to field phone calls from people who heard *somewhere* that "cryotherapy cures cancer" or "cold exposure makes you smarter" or "cryo can make you young again," and these ideas aren't just unproven, they're exceptionally unlikely.

All that brings us back to Payton. Thankfully, he was in pretty good health and wasn't looking for a "miracle cure" for anything. But he had heard a lot of different claims about cryotherapy—some well supported by science and others a bit outlandish—and was intrigued by the myriad possibilities.

"At the same time, I went in a little skeptical," he said. "I'll try anything once. And maybe if the science suggests that it's something I need to do a few times to feel an effect, I'll try that too, but if I'm doing something to my body, I do want proof that it's working for me."

Payton found a Restore center next to a gym near his home. "I went in, did the thing, and left," he recalled. "And I know some people say it was immediately transformative, but for me it was interesting and I definitely felt some adrenaline, but I didn't walk away going 'OK, I'm hooked.'"

But then something transformative really did happen. "I went to bed that night and had the best night of sleep of my life," he said. "I mean, I woke up feeling like I'd experienced sleep in a way that I'd never known was possible."

Payton's sleep tracker confirmed what he suspected: Ordinarily he would experience two or three periods of deep sleep and two or three periods of REM in about seven hours of sleep each night, with at least one fitful wakeup in the middle of the night that usually lasted 20 to 30 minutes. That night he had "gone deep" four times, ascended into REM three times, and remained in a state of slumber for eight hours total without any lengthy period of wakefulness until the sun came up the next morning.

Then, something else happened. For years, Payton had been doing the same set of exercises, "just push-ups and stuff like that," he said. "I always tried to do as many as possible in a set amount of time. And the next time I did that, I destroyed my max in almost every exercise. It was insane."

He pored over his health journal. "I thought, what did I eat? What supplement did I take? But the only change was that I'd done cryo and gotten that amazing night of sleep as a result," he said.

What Payton learned on that day was that even though he had a lot of tailwinds working for him, he'd never had the benefit of a full wind behind his back. "It was just that little investment in trying something new that told me I really could do more," he said. "I could sleep better and that meant I could exercise better. I knew what my actual personal best was, which gave me something to work harder toward achieving and again and again—and the cool thing is that exercising toward a goal like that has the benefit of leaving you really ready for sleep at the end of the day, so even if it has been a few days since I've gotten to go to cryo I still sleep really well."

But sauna and cryo aren't the only therapies that have a huge impact on sleep.

Hyperbaric Sleep

It's not as futuristically sleek as we might see in a sci-fi movie, but a room full of people undergoing mild hyperbaric oxygen therapy always reminds us of the "hibernation room" from *Passengers,* the 2016 film starring Chris Pratt and Jennifer Lawrence as space travelers who are awakened early from their century-long voyage to another planet.

It's not just the size and shape of the mHbOT pods that makes this connection so tangible. It's also the fact that, quite frequently, everybody inside them is peacefully snoozing, as if they could stay that way on a long journey between stars.

If you've ever taken a long nap during the day, then found yourself struggling to get to sleep at night, you're not alone. People who feel they have no choice but to nap during the day are less likely to sleep well at night, which leaves them more tired during the day, which makes them more likely to need a nap—and onward this vicious cycle goes.[10] And so it might seem to stand to reason that people who fall asleep while undergoing a session of HbOT or mHbOT might also have trouble getting back to sleep that night, but that's not what happens. In fact, one of the commonly reported effects of hyperbaric therapy is better sleep.

As is common, the initial and most comprehensive evidence for this association came in studies of people suffering from other medical challenges. HbOT has been shown to be especially effective for sleep disorders in children with cerebral palsy,[11] for US armed service members with mild traumatic brain injuries,[12] and in people recovering from a stroke.[13]

Why does oxygen treatment seem to work so well to promote better sleep for people with such a wide variety of conditions? Foremost, it's because circulating blood levels of O_2 play a crucial role in healthy brain function, as has been demonstrated by Canadian neuroscientists who used brain scans to show that rats who are brought into a state of hyperoxia are more likely to fall into the patterns crucial to setting the pace for the smooth and steady transitions between deep and REM indicative of restorative rest.[14]

But researchers associated with the delightfully named Clinical Center for Pleasant Sleep in Tokyo have pointed to another crucial piece of this puzzle. After demonstrating the significant impact HbOT has on helping patients with a wide variety of instigating conditions get a better night of rest, they noted that while oxygen might indeed play a role in promoting restful brain patterns, "we cannot exclude the possibility that this improvement is mediated by the alleviation of their original symptoms, primarily pain."[15]

Of course, it's most likely that hyperbaric oxygen plays a multifaceted role in promoting sleep. But from our perspective, the underlying reasons—while fascinating—are less important than the life-changing results. We've seen those results at Restore centers across the nation, and as is the case for so many of the interventions we've discussed in this book, you don't have to have a medical condition that is adversely impacting your sleep in order to benefit from the whole-body boost of oxygen that comes from hyperbaric therapy.

Restore client Bei is a great example. Bei was in her late 30s and, she says, in the best shape of her life when she first used hyperbaric oxygen. "I was on vacation in Mexico and my girlfriends and I found out about a center where six people can go into the chamber together," she said. "And when I got there and saw it, I almost ran away because I got panicky about being locked in that thing, especially since there were two guys they put in our group who we didn't even know, but I did relax a bit once it started."

The next morning, Bei woke up feeling so rested that she felt like she was on another planet. "Part of me was like, 'Well, yeah, I'm on vacation, so I should be feeling this way,' but then again I've gone on lots of vacations and never felt like that before," she recalled.

A few weeks after returning to her home in Denver, Bei decided she'd like to try it again. "There wasn't really a reason for me to do it," she said. "I wasn't sick or injured. But that first experience had been so interesting, and I was attracted to the idea that maybe it had something to do with how rested I felt, so I was just curious." But, she said, she didn't want to be locked into a "hard chamber" again, so she opted to try mHbOT.

"That night I had another amazing night of sleep," she said. "It's a little hard to explain, but I felt like I'd been rebooted, where just one good night of sleep led to another, and so on like that, and all that better sleep was helping me stay focused during the day and have more energy for my friends and family."

"I felt like I'd been rebooted, where just one good night of sleep led to another, and so on like that."

Bei now does one mHbOT session every two weeks. "Fourteen or fifteen days sort of seems like the sweet spot where I start to feel the momentum begin to shift a little," she said. "Then I do one session and it puts me right back into that rhythm where my sleep is just really good, night after night."

Inherent in Bei's hyperbaric routine is that she didn't treat this therapy as a "one and done" experience. It's something she knows that she'll be doing for a long time to come as part of a sustain practice of hyper wellness.

Sleep Is Something We Must Keep Working At

Nobody expects one day of exercise to result in a longer and healthier life. And nobody thinks a week of dieting is going to lower their long-term risk of obesity and other diseases. These are things we must keep working on, day after day, for our entire lives.

Sleep is the same way. While it's clear to us that many people can jump-start a healthy rhythm with interventions like cryo, sauna, and hyperbaric therapy, those things alone are unlikely to help you stay inside the virtuous cycle if you're not pursuing good "sleep hygiene," the practices that experts like Chris Winter and Matthew Walker say are the essential starting places for a lifetime of better sleep.

The great news is that none of these practices require access to a place like Restore. So, as we've been saying repeatedly in this book, even though we absolutely want people to feel that our studios are an important part of their wellness journey, that's not where the journey absolutely must begin. Much to the contrary, for most people a more restful, restorative, and wellness-inducing night of sleep is just a few easy lifestyle changes away.

The first of these changes is hard for many people: committing to "screenless evenings," just like Becca did, thus eliminating the blue light exposure that triggers your brain to produce signaling chemicals associated with being awake (and delays the production of chemicals that help bring you toward sleep). If you must be exposed to a screen late into the night, screen filters or orange-hued glasses have been shown to be helpful,[16] but it's important to note that these interventions generally won't help you achieve the same level of sleep that you would get if you had no screen exposure at all before bedtime. For this reason, it can be helpful to develop an evening hobby that can be done without a screen and, better yet, in diminishing quantities of light as the hour gets later, like reading physical books, writing letters, assembling models, listening to music or audio books, or working on puzzles. Remember, your body is the product of millions of years of evolution that programmed your brain to move toward rest when the sun went down. Barely a century has gone by since ubiquitous electrical lighting threw off those patterns. So, the closer you can get to natural diurnality, the better. For this same reason, increasing your exposure to light first thing in the morning can help bring you into alignment with the natural circadian rhythm that regulate a healthy pattern of sleep and rest. (We'll discuss the role of light further in chapter 8.)

It probably goes without saying that caffeine and other stimulants aren't conducive to these patterns, but few people realize how powerful a cup of coffee or can of soda can be on sleep even when you drink it early in the day. Caffeine is metabolized by an enzyme encoded by a gene known as CYP1A2, and about half of the population has a variant in this gene that makes them less able to efficiently process that stimulant. These slow metabolizers tend to be at greater risk for a variety of conditions, especially heart attacks[17]—likely because they aren't getting as much restorative, disease-fighting, wellness-inducing sleep as a result of their reduced ability to process this stimulant. Thus, for most people, caffeine in the late afternoon can disturb nighttime slumber, but for some people, caffeine at *any* time at all can be harmful. Unless you happen to know your CYP1A2 status, it can be helpful to assume that caffeine isn't doing you any favors.

Because alcohol is a depressant, a lot of people assume it's helpful for sleep. That's not true. The research suggests that while alcohol *might* help you get to sleep, it's also likely to interfere with the production of chemicals that help you stay asleep and fall into a smooth, peaceful flow through each stage of sleep that is indicative of restorative sleep. Yet most people drink exclusively in the evenings, so they are interfering with their ability to get a restorative night of rest. This is one of the reasons why—while it's not popular to point out—the science is clear that there's *no* level of alcohol consumption that is beneficial for our long-term wellness.[18]

Population health investigations have shown a negative relationship between exposure to air pollution and the ability of people to get healthy sleep[19]—and given the vital role of oxygen in promoting deep sleep, this makes plenty of sense. If you live in an area with excessive air pollution (and relative to the air we evolved to breathe, that really is just about every populated place on the planet) you may benefit from a high-efficiency particulate (HEPA) air filter.

The toxic particulates in our air are only the most obvious form of pollution, though. There's another pollutant that should be equally noted: noise. The noise outside your home—from airplanes overhead to cars driving by to neighbors who like to play music late into the night—might be so constant that you don't even think about it anymore, but studies have shown that it's a significant source of elevated stress hormones that can cause metabolic destabilization and mental health problems, again likely in association with the impact that noise has on interfering with people's ability to get to sleep and stay asleep.[20] For these reasons, investing in a pair of earplugs designed for sleep can offer an immediate return on investment in the quality of sleep you get each night.[21]

We could write an entire book on sleep hygiene—but Winter, Walker, and others have that covered. It suffices to say that while sleep is an element of wellness just about everyone needs to work hard at, it's not an element of wellness that is hard to impact with small decisions that build greater capacity, which can then be invested into other decisions that build even greater capacity. And all of us already have some tailwinds working in our favor, because even if we sleep poorly, we do ultimately sleep. Our bodies demand it of us. The trick to better sleep is fulfilling that demand with increasing regularity and rhythm.

chapter 8

light

Like tens of millions of other people, Mandy Erickson spent the first few months of the COVID-19 pandemic working from home.

That transition was hard for a lot of people, with many at-home workers complaining of exhaustion, fitful nights of sleep, immense stress, and constantly feeling as though they were getting sick—even when they knew they weren't infected because, of course, they'd been away from people that whole time!

This wasn't just the case in the United States. One 2021 study from researchers in Portugal and Switzerland demonstrated that those who worked from home in the first phase of the pandemic were more likely to suffer from depression, anxiety, and sleeping difficulties.[1] Those findings were backed in the following year by public health experts in the United Kingdom whose research demonstrated an increase in the same conditions, especially if those workers already had an underlying mental health issue.[2]

These experiences and fears could have been tied to the stress that came along with the pandemic itself, but research has suggested there may have been something additional and perhaps even more pernicious at play for workers who were unable to go into the office. It might also explain why, even though she was subject to the same stresses as so many others were during this time, Erickson managed quite well. Writing about her experience several months into the pandemic, the associate editor at the Stanford School of Medicine marveled that, for some reason, "I'm sleeping fine and feeling little stress while sheltering in place."[3]

The secret to her smooth transition to working from home may have been her dog—a Chihuahua–Jack Russell terrier mix she walks every day before work. Researchers have long known that dog ownership provides a huge boost in mental and physical health, and the assumption has been that the exercise and companionship dogs bring to their owners is a powerful combination for improved wellness. That's probably true, to some extent. But neurobiologist Andrew Huberman, who also works at Stanford, thinks there may have been a hidden factor at play in Erickson's situation: the natural sunlight she was getting each morning when she walked her dog.

In recent years, Huberman has become a zealous evangelist for daily exposure to morning sunlight, which increases the release of cortisol, a hormone that drives the feeling of wakefulness and helps regulate immunity and metabolism. And what happens when people leave their homes to go to work in the morning? They get a dose of morning light. Millions of people who were no longer leaving their homes to go to work weren't getting this "morning kick," but Erickson was because each morning, right after breakfast, she took her dog for a walk—just as she had every day before the pandemic.

This daily dose of morning light likely kept Erickson's circadian rhythms flowing just as they always had been, while "optic flow"—the movement of homes, trees, cars, and all the other things they passed when Erickson and her dog left their home in the morning—quieted some of the circuits that create stress.

It doesn't take a pandemic to screw up the rhythms of light and darkness that have mediated animal behavior since long before humans existed. Artificial light, backlit screens, schedules that have some of us waking up at 9 a.m. on one day and 4 a.m. the next, and the movement we see on television and computer screens even though we're sitting perfectly still all wreak havoc on these rhythms. As a result, many people have been out of sync with this ancient signal for years or even decades. And some people have *never* been in sync!

But if anything speaks to the power of light in our lives, it's this: For many people, a healthful pattern can be reset in just a few days and, in fact, some people can get back into rhythm in a single day. That's because, in most places where people live, the sun's reliable movement around Earth, plus deeply reinforced genetic programming, has conditioned humans to actively *pursue* circadian balance, feeling more drawn to sleep at night even when they are rested, compelled to wake in the morning even when they haven't gotten enough sleep. Indeed, this is why we experience jet lag as our bodies adjust to what we are internally wired to crave at certain times of the day, what we're getting, and what we actually need to function.

Many people have been out of sync with this ancient signal for years or even decades. And some people have never been in sync!

Whenever possible, the effort to utilize this underappreciated tailwind of wellness should start with either getting outside or spending a few minutes in a sunlit window each morning. Even on overcast days, cloud-penetrating ultraviolet rays are still present, and these wavelengths have been shown to be powerful for the regulation of cortisol and other biochemical mediators of wellness.[4]

Twilight is equally important. The pineal gland, a small hormone-secreting structure at the center of our brains, is designed to respond to waning sunlight with the production of melatonin, which in addition to making us feel sleepy also has antioxidant and anti-inflammatory properties. When we help this part of our brain do its job by weaning ourselves off unnatural sources of light as we approach our bedtimes, we are opening our sails to this tailwind.

But let's also be realistic here: Few people have the luxury of waking and returning to slumber with the rising and setting of the sun, day after day throughout their lives. Hundreds of millions of people live in very northerly and southerly latitudes, with very long days in one season and very long nights in another. Billions do work that requires them to rise before or go to bed after the sun crosses the sky above them. The electronic screens that surround us are sometimes not something we are willing or able to ignore.

So, we cannot pretend that integrating this element of hyper wellness into our lives is easy. But we cannot ignore it, either: We have to "see the light."

Or perhaps it would be better to say "We have to see the *lights*," for light isn't a singular thing. Just as medications derived from different plants produce different biophysical effects, various parts of the infrared, visual, and ultraviolet spectrum have different impacts on our health. Many of these effects can be felt right away, thus accentuating the feel-better-do-more cycle that leads to hyper wellness. Once this is made clear, it becomes easy to see all the things that can be done to use light to enhance energy, thus growing capacity, leading us ever closer to the goal of hyper wellness.

The Unseen Spectrum

By a strict and classical definition, light is the spectrum of radiation that can be *seen*. And since members of our species have always tended to think in anthropocentric ways, light has historically been described as the natural force that stimulates *human* sight, making things visible to *our* eyes.

This is a limiting construct. There are bands of light that our eyes cannot interpret but that are nonetheless there. Some species of snakes can see infrared light. Some amphibians, insects, and fish can, too. Many of these same animals can also see on the other end of the spectrum, too, via UV-sensitive photoreceptors, and so do some nonhuman mammals, including cats, dogs, mice, pigs, cows, and even reindeer. And whether visible to humans or not, all these parts of the spectrum may have an impact on our state of wellness.

This is not a new concept. In ancient Egypt, for instance, healers practiced a form of therapy in which exposure to certain colors—literally the reflection of visible light from different surfaces into the red-, blue-, and green-sensing cones of our retinas—were used to treat a variety of ailments. That might sound absurd, but there's substantial modern research that demonstrates that visible color can impact people's moods and states of mental health. Whether because of social conditioning or innate neurological programming, for instance, bright red colors often provoke anger or arousal, while blue incites focus and alertness.[5] What's more, in pharaonic times, there was no conceptual separation between diseases of the body and diseases of the mind—Egyptian medical texts advised physicians to treat mental disorders with the same kinds of therapies they would apply to somatic ailments.[6] Thus, if these healers recognized that certain colors had an impact on the part of wellness we now consider to be "mental," it would have been logical to assume there could be an impact on the side of health we now consider to be "physical" as well.

It's likely there was even earlier and widespread recognition that all parts of the visible spectrum—that is to say sunlight in general—can be beneficial to a person's wellness. Parents have probably been telling moody children to "go outside and play" since the days of our cave-dwelling ancestors, but one of the earliest surviving texts that relates this dictum as generalized health advice comes from the ancient Ayurvedic physician Charaka, who is thought to have lived about 2,000 years ago, and who prescribed "exposure to the sun" to treat a variety of ailments, including fever, nausea, heart disease, and cholera.

In more modern times, the idea that sunlight could be restorative to those suffering from illness and injury was given a big boost by Florence Nightingale, who, while serving as a hospital supervisor during the Crimean War in the 1850s, instructed the nurses under her command to position patients close to windows, which offered the benefits of fresh air and direct sunlight.[7]

Nightingale has been immortalized as "The Lady with the Lamp," which is important in historical context, as electric lights would remain an uncommon feature of society for another half century. This meant that no one could have known much about which parts of the visible and invisible light spectrum were therapeutic, since all those parts came together in the form of the sunlight and all the things that reflected it, and little could be done to filter the spectrum in the controlled ways necessary to experiment with individual bands of light.

In the wake of work by inventors like Thomas Edison and Nikola Tesla to make electricity safer and more accessible in the late 1800s, though, a pioneering Danish physician named Niels Finsen was able to build and use a filtered electric light to research the impacts of different wavelengths on different diseases, using short wavelength light (perceptible to humans as violet or purple light) to treat lupus and longer wavelength (perceptible as red light) to treat smallpox lesions in experiments for which he was awarded the Nobel Prize in Medicine in 1903.

With such an auspicious beginning—and more than a hundred years of time separating our modern world from Finsen's early work in phototherapy—it might seem strange that light exposure doesn't play a more ubiquitous role in modern medicine. That's in no small part a result of the fact that many of the conditions that Finsen and others were seeking to cure in the early 1900s were acute infectious diseases—the sorts that, as it turned out, were effectively defeated with antibiotics and other single-target drugs. With those weapons at hand, doctors and researchers had little incentive to dive into what then seemed to be less-effective cures, so much of the promising initial progress related to phototherapy stalled out for decades to come. Thus, like so many of the other therapies we've discussed in this book, phototherapy was effectively sidelined and even derided as pseudoscience.

It would take another half century—and some significant advancements in our understanding of the ultraviolet and infrared parts of the light spectrum—before phototherapy would regain even a small foothold in mainstream medical research when it was shown to have applications in dermatological care and, as many people who have had a jaundiced baby know, for the treatment of hyperbilirubinemia. Today, emerging peer-reviewed scientific evidence demonstrates that—just as our ancestors suspected many thousands of years ago—different wavelengths of light do indeed have different beneficial effects on our health, and phototherapy is now used in ophthalmology, dermatology, cardiology, and rheumatology; for chronic pain control, cancer care, mental health treatment, and heart care; and for the treatment of neurological diseases such as Parkinson's disease, traumatic brain injury, and multiple sclerosis.[8]

Emerging peer-reviewed scientific evidence demonstrates that—just as our ancestors suspected many thousands of years ago—different wavelengths of light do indeed have different beneficial effects on our health.

We're still only just beginning to understand what different frequencies can do to modulate human health, and even further behind in understanding the mechanisms that drive these impacts. But Michael Hamblin, who spent decades studying photobiomodulation at Massachusetts General Hospital and Harvard Medical School, has suggested that the first step in understanding the biomolecular underpinnings of these reactions is to better understand chromophores, molecules that absorb particular wavelengths of visible light. Traditionally, these molecules were thought to play a role only in the generation of color, but Hamblin and others have pointed out that when a cellular chromophore is doing its job, the energy being taken in and stored must go *somewhere* and do *something*.

Hamblin has noted, for instance, that red and near-infrared light seems to be well absorbed by a certain chromophore that can be prodigiously found on the outer membranes of mitochondria, which exist inside nearly every cell in the human body—including in the skin, which in addition to being the largest organ of the body is also, and obviously, the most easily affected by light. The chromophore at play here is called cytochrome C oxidase and, true to its role as an oxidase, its job is to mediate the transfer of electrons into molecular oxygen. But, in reaction to red light absorption, it has also been shown to impact the production of adenosine triphosphate, or ATP, which is essential for converting food into energy in the human body. Blue and green light, on the other hand, may be best absorbed by chromophores known as opsins, flavins, and cryptochromes. When opsins absorb light, the result is a change in the shape and formation of proteins, a stimulus that prompts a biochemical signaling cascade that changes how messages are relayed and amplified from cell to cell across the body. Flavins, meanwhile, can be "excited" by light in a way that instigates a reduction in the oxidation state of molecules throughout the body. And cryptochromes are photoreceptors that regulate how light impacts circadian rhythm.[9]

These are the sorts of reactions that we are used to seeing in the human body as a result of the ingestion of drugs—and any pharmaceutical with these sorts of effects would be exceedingly well studied for its potential impacts on human health. And yet when it comes to the potential for light to help move us further in our journey toward hyper wellness, we've still only touched the very edge of the rainbow.

Thankfully, though, that's changing. You might even say it's changing at the speed of light.

Moods and Mental Health

Larissa's path to red light therapy—and her first step onto the virtuous cycle—started with a trip to Sin City.

"We weren't trying to be healthy, we were just trying to keep raging," the disabilities case manager and Air Force wife said as she recalled getting her first IV drip at a hotel on the Las Vegas Strip. "It was super pricey, but it was obvious that it helped. We weren't hung over. We weren't tired. It was sort of crazy how much it worked."

That's why, shortly after returning home from Vegas, Larissa found her way to a Restore studio near her home. "But of course when you come in you see right away that it's not just IV drips," she said. "There were all these other options. And it's fun to try everything out, at least a few times, to see how it works for you."

That's how Larissa found her way to red light therapy, also known as photobiomodulation therapy, which employs red and near-infrared light sources to induce physiological reactions, just as Niels Finsen was seeking to do more than a century ago (albeit in significantly more modern, technologically sophisticated, and controlled settings).

There are many versions of red and near-infrared therapy, including wands that can be waved across the body, blankets that can be draped over someone as they are lying down, small T-shaped contraptions drawn over the skin like a safety razor, and even quasi-futuristic helmets that look like something from an old Buck Rogers movie or a Daft Punk concert. After investigating all these options and more, taking a long and deep dive into the available research, and consulting with our medical advisory board, Restore opted for a relatively straightforward approach to broad *exposure*. At Restore studios across the nation, clients step out of their clothes in private rooms where they stand in front of large panels with thousands of powerful light-emitting diodes, which create a bright and warm environment that many describe as "bathing in red light." A typical session takes about 15 minutes.

"It's become an absolute must for me and I try to do it at least every week," Larissa said. "When it's gloomy outside or cold I do red light treatment, and I've noticed a huge impact on the way I feel, and especially when it comes to anxiety, it just soothes me."

She's not alone. One of the first modern study of the impacts of red-light photobiomodulation therapy on human mood came in 2009, when a team of researchers from Harvard University and several nearby hospitals ran a pilot study investigating the impact of red light therapy on patients with depression and anxiety, and found that a single treatment resulted in a decrease of the patients' symptoms for two weeks.[10] In 2015, a separate group of researchers from Boston and New York demonstrated that a series of six treatments could be even more effective.[11]

As is the case for so many of the other therapies discussed in this book so far, the impact on the mental health and moods of people who are not symptomatically suffering or classically diagnosed hasn't been well studied. Alas, most research is focused on whether a treatment or therapy helps sick people get well and doesn't bother to examine what keeps well people from getting sick!

Larissa's friend Ken was a part of that same trip to Vegas and also got hooked on the Restore therapies shortly after returning home. He doesn't deal with any known underlying mental health conditions, but he can also attest to how he feels when he walks out of a red light booth.

"It's remarkable to me," the retired businessman and amateur poet from Idaho said. "I come out and I feel like I'm half my mass. It feels like all my cells are alive. All my cells are just buzzing." And that feeling of enhanced energy lasts for days afterward—enhancing his capacity to take other steps that lead to an even longer-lasting effect.

"It's hard to explain," Ken said, "but I guess the easiest way to describe it is that I just feel happier and more positive about life, and when you feel that way it's just easier to keep the good times rolling."

Brain Health

If photobiomodulation can positively impact mental health, then the next best place to look for beneficial applications would be other forms of brain health. Indeed, that's what researchers have been studying since the mid-2000s.

In more than a dozen animal studies and at least a half dozen human studies that have been conducted since then, researchers have found that various modes of photobiomodulation therapies can be effective in mitigating the long-term damages associated with traumatic brain injury, or TBI. Among the most compelling of these studies was a report published in 2018 describing the impact of pulsed red and near-infrared light therapy on a group of US military veterans. The chronic nature of their diagnosis is telling: These were individuals who had been suffering from TBI for at least 18 months, and for whom any improvements in their conditions under standard methods of care had either stalled out or had never materialized to begin with. But when doctors exposed those patients to 400 red and infrared light emitting diodes for 20 minutes, three times per week, for six weeks, something astounding happened: a sudden improvement in cerebral blood flow, brain activity, and brain function.[12] And while this was a small study, its findings align with several other initial studies that have investigated the impacts of photobiomodulation therapy and TBI, which has led researchers to wonder about the mechanisms at play past the now well-accepted understanding that light at different wavelengths can impact chromophores.

One promising hypothesis comes from Brazilian researchers who have observed that photobiomodulation therapy in rats can slow the production of cytokines,[13] small proteins known to promote inflammation—which has been shown to be a contributing factor in clinical and functional outcomes for TBI patients.[14] Meanwhile, a joint team of neurologists from the Medical College of Wisconsin and Ohio State University have shown that photobiomodulation may increase mitochondrial function,[15] thus potentially increasing the vast amounts of energy needed to heal the most energy-hungry organ in the human body.

It's likely no coincidence that inflammation and mitochondrial production appear to be significant factors in the development and escalation of Alzheimer's disease as well,[16] and this might be why multiple studies have shown that high-intensity near-infrared therapy has been shown to reduce amyloid beta plaques—a hallmark pathology for dementia—in the brains of mice with a rodent version of Alzheimer's.[17]

Michael Hamblin, the photobiomodulation expert mentioned earlier, has been further compelled by studies showing that infrared, near-infrared, and red light therapy can improve metabolism, blood flow, neuroprotective functioning, and the creation of new neurons—all biological functions generally diminished in Alzheimer's patients. "The fact that photobiomodulation therapy may produce a large range of beneficial changes in the brain, and is without any major side effects, suggests it should be more widely tested," he wrote in 2019.

Slowly, that's happening. But there are many who, in the meantime, aren't content to sit around and wait.

Among those who are proactively using red light therapy in this way is Miguel, a carpentry shop manager who, like an increasing number of people around the world, decided to have his genome sequenced for the purpose of informing lifestyle decisions that can impact his health. In doing so, Miguel learned that he is an inheritor of a form of a gene associated with about half of all cases of Alzheimer's, a variant known as APOE-e4. "We've lost people on both sides of my family to Alzheimer's, so I guess it wasn't a surprise, but it still took me some time to process," the Nashville resident explained. "I knew even before I got sequenced that just because you have a gene doesn't mean you're completely destined for some specific outcome, but the deck gets stacked in a way, and I knew that it was going to be really important for me to do what I could to level the odds in favor of good brain health."

For Miguel, that meant switching to a Mediterranean diet, which many studies have shown to be associated with a reduced risk of the development and progression of Alzheimer's.[18] He was also compelled by research into how cognitive training can improve the ability of neural networks to reorganize over time, a function know as neuroplasticity that has been shown to be drastically reduced in dementia patients.[19] In light of this knowledge, he began participating in a daily "brain training" program.[20] And after watching a video in which Alzheimer's prevention advocate Dale Bredesen and photobiomodulation pioneer Marvin Berman discussed the potential power of near-infrared light on preventing, delaying, and potentially even reversing some symptoms of Alzheimer's, Miguel began making weekly visits to a Restore studio near his home to, as he calls it, "hang out on Mars."

"I knew that it was going to be really important for me to do what I could to level the odds in favor of good brain health."

"That's what it feels like to me," he laughed. "It's sort of an otherworldly experience. I turn on some brown noise on my phone and close my eyes and time slows down. I don't meditate, exactly, but it feels meditative."

Is it working to counteract the increased risks that Miguel faces as a carrier of the APOE-e4 variant? That's something he will never know. Even if he someday winds up with Alzheimer's, it will be impossible to know whether any of the preventative strategies he tried slowed the onset or progression. And even if he never gets Alzheimer's, he won't be able to say that his luck would have been different if he'd done nothing at all. But acknowledging these truths is not at all the same as saying that Miguel isn't bettering the odds in his favor, because he is, thanks in no small part to the things he absolutely does know red light therapy is doing—because some benefits are palpable *right away*.

"I usually go to Restore around lunch and always on that afternoon I notice a big difference in my mental clarity," he said. "And always on that night, I get amazingly good sleep, and that's not just speculation. I can see it in my sleep tracker. I'm going deeper, getting longer REM, and all that stuff."

As a result, Miguel said, he has the energy to exercise more the next day. And since scores of studies have shown that people who are physically active have a significantly lowered risk of developing Alzheimer's disease,[21] Miguel is improving his odds of maintaining strong brain function through exercise as well.

"There's something else about all this that's a little hard to explain, but I definitely feel in my life," he said. "It's this thing where, at first when I learned about my genetic risk, I felt really unlucky. And then as I started doing more and more to try to prevent it, and those things all started to build on one another—like how red light helps me sleep and good sleep helps me get more exercise—there's a point when I realized that I was doing everything I could, and so I'm not stressing out about it anymore."

Stress itself is a significant predictor of Alzheimer's risk.[22] So, as Miguel found himself at peace with his risk as a result of what he was doing to fight that risk, he was lowering the risk even more!

So far, we've mostly been discussing the impact of light on various facets of brain health. But that's not the only place in our bodies where light therapy can help set us on a path toward hyper wellness.

More Than Skin Deep

Nachelle's first psoriasis flare-up happened when she was 17.

"I went on a camping trip with some friends and I got bitten so many times on the first night by mosquitos," the native of Salem, Oregon, recalled. "We were supposed to be camping for three days, but the next morning I woke up and it was like my skin was on fire, and I knew I needed to get home."

The drive took about two hours and, by the time she got back to her town, her skin had turned bright red and was cracking all over. "I was so scared that I called my mom and she gave me the address to the doctor's office," she said. "So, I drove straight there."

The doctor on duty told Nachelle that the mosquitoes had likely triggered a psoriasis flare-up, and over the next few years it became clear that any time Nachelle suffered from even a small cut, prick, scrape, or bug bite, it would trigger a new buildup of psoriasis plaques.

Topical and oral medications didn't seem to do much to help. But the next year, when Nachelle arrived as a freshman at Portland State University, a nurse at the student health center asked if she'd ever tried light therapy.

Nachelle was skeptical at first. "My mom is a chemist, and my dad is a physiology teacher," she said. "So, I grew up to be focused on science, and that just sounded—well, in my home the word we'd use was *woo-woo*—but I also was taught to look for evidence, so that's what I did."

She didn't have to look hard. Going back to the 1970s, dermatologists have been employing a combinatory treatment in which a patient either takes an oral drug or bathes in water that includes a solution of psoralens—a drug that modifies how skin cells react to light—and then undergoes UV light exposure. While this technique, which is called PUVA, has been known to be effective in many patients for decades, it hasn't been clear why it worked until more recently, when researchers demonstrated that the treatment appears to decrease the expression of several inflammatory cytokines[23]—the same kinds of proteins that we mentioned earlier in connection to traumatic brain injury.

Although this has a long history of effectiveness, it's also time-consuming. The initial treatment phase often requires two or three visits to a clinic each week for up to four months, and then "maintenance visits" that occur monthly or even more—often for the rest of a person's life. Nachelle was more than willing to give it a try, though, and found a clinic at Oregon Health & Science University that could take her as a new patient.

"I really started looking forward to it," she said. "The people at the clinic were really nice, and I think that even before I noticed a difference in my skin, there was a difference in my mood, and I probably looked really silly because I think I was riding the bus with a funny grin on my face whenever I was going to the clinic."

Indeed, multiple studies have shown that ultraviolet light can spark a chain of biochemical reactions that can impact a person's mood for the better.[24] What really got Nachelle feeling better about her life, though, was when her PUVA sessions started improving the appearance of her skin.

"There was a big difference," she said. "But it wasn't perfect, and that's one of the things you have to come to terms with when you're dealing with psoriasis—or at least something I had to accept. It was a lot better, but it wasn't a silver bullet."

But once Nachelle's eyes had been opened to the power of light to impact her skin health, she began investigating other ways the light spectrum might help her deal with her skin condition. That's when she learned that while UV light therapy—which focuses on the "bluer" end of the spectrum—had a longer history, some researchers and patients have found red light therapy to be effective as well.[25] "There are a lot of reported side effects for PUVA, and I was lucky that I never had any of those, but even if I did, I think it would have been worth it to me," Nachelle said. "But red light therapy doesn't include any drugs, and it doesn't have any reported side effects, so it made sense to me to at least try it out."

The bus ride to the closest Restore studio took just a bit longer than the one that got her to her PUVA clinic, but it turned out to be well worth the time. "I'd just study for an hour on the bus, hop off, go get my 15 minutes of red light, and then be back on campus an hour later," she said. "And it was totally something that I looked forward to, just like with the UV therapy, because it really did feel like it made me happier."

It also seemed to clear up what PUVA didn't. Today, Nachelle supplements her monthly maintenance session of PUVA with twice-monthly red light sessions, "and now my skin is so healthy that when I do see a patch of red or dry skin it actually surprises me. That used to be just my normal experience and now it's something I hardly deal with at all."

The importance of these sorts of transformations can't be understated. By some estimates, the life expectancy of individuals with psoriasis is up to 10 years shorter than the general public. It's not hard to understand why this might be. Our skin, after all, is the largest organ in our bodies, and the one that serves a protective function for everything else. When skin itself is under duress, it cannot serve this function as well. That's likely one of the key reasons that people with psoriasis are at a higher risk of cardiovascular disease, diabetes, lymphoma, and accelerated aging.[26]

It's also why skin health is important for *everyone*. The more we can protect this organ, the more it can protect us.

Every part of our skin is important. The thin top layer, the epidermis, acts as a protective barrier and continually replaces old cells with new cells, leaving us with a brand new outer layer every month or so. The also-thin bottom layer, the fatty hypodermis, cushions our muscles and bones against impact injuries and plays an important role in body temperature regulation. But it's the middle layer, the dermis, that makes up 90 percent of our skin's thickness. And 70 percent of this layer is made up of collagen, which is essential for skin strength and resilience. Thus, while there is no element of skin we should ignore, if you want the greatest "bang for your buck" in terms of holistic wellness, collagen is a good place to start.

Supplemental collagen is a global industry worth billions of dollars each year that many analysts believe will increase severalfold in the coming decades. But supplements are just one research-backed way to potentially increase skin collagen.[27] Foods such as fish, poultry, eggs, and legumes, which are high in glycine, proline, and hydroxyproline—the amino acids that make up collagen—are another. And, as you might have now guessed, light therapy is yet another.

For many decades, dermatologists have employed scaled rating systems to assess patient skin health, using reference photos of patients in different stages of the progression of a specific skin condition. Among the most common of these systems—and one often used as a proxy for collagen health—is the Modified Fitzpatrick Wrinkle Scale, which is based on a series of reference photographs used by trained assessors to evaluate the lines that form on people's faces with aging, particularly as the result of a loss of structural collagen. Using this system—and employing three independent physicians who were blinded to the clinical patient data and could see only the photos—a team of researchers from Germany found in 2014 that red light therapy was effective at smoothing wrinkles, presumably as a result of a boost in collagen health. Unsatisfied with that supposition, the researchers also took a series of ultrasonic photographs of the study participants, who were treated twice a week with 30 treatments in total. The results were striking. In the ultrasonic images, black and green areas represent a lack of collagen, while yellow and red regions show more robust collagen health. On the first day of the experiment, one image of a 46-year-old female participant's skin revealed mostly black with flecks of green—and just a few dots of yellow and red. In a second image, taken after the 30th round of red light treatment, the yellow and red areas had exploded, with several thick layers of healthy collagen apparent in the photograph.[28]

Results like that have prompted some to see light therapy as a panacea. That's unlikely. What we do believe, however, is that there are a lot of areas of health in which light may play a vital role—but health researchers are still in the early stages of identifying what those areas are.

Muscle Recovery and Athletic Performance

No one yet knows what bands of infrared, visible, or ultraviolet light are right for every person in every state of health—and anyone who claims to have already discovered the "perfect" wavelength for human health and performance is a liar.

In fact, even when it comes to a specific goal, like athletic performance, the available data is mixed. In general, it can certainly be said that red and near infrared therapy has been shown in various studies to delay the onset of muscle soreness after exercise, improve repetitions and contractions when used before exercise, and positively impact the presence of several biomarkers in the bloodstream associated with exercise. But the dozens of studies conducted to explore this topic have all been completed in different ways, with different modes of irradiation, different exposure times, different types of exercise, and different participant groups. So when a team of researchers from Massachusetts General Hospital, Harvard Medical School, and Brazil's Sacred Heart University gathered all the studies they could find in search of "a final prescription of the exact doses of light for general use" in athletic performance, they came up empty. "There are more positive effects in favor of photobiomodulation than there are conflicting results or negative results," the researchers reported in 2016, adding that "if all the positive results achieved in laboratory settings go on to demonstrate comparable improvements in sports performance in the real world, photobiomodulation will become very popular mainly amongst high level athletes."[29]

They were certainly right about that. We've seen it firsthand in studios across the United States, where high school, college, and professional athletes come for pre- and post-training red light therapy sessions.

In one study, an international team of researchers worked together to pore over the performance, biometric data, and epigenetic data of two men—one of whom was treated with photobiomodulation therapy while, unbeknownst to either person, the other went through a similar-looking therapy that used lights that looked the same but did not produce the same infrared wavelength. Each person did the same combination of weight-training exercises three times a week for 12 weeks, and muscle biopsies, magnetic resonance imaging, max lifts, and fatigue resistance tests were conducted before and after the experiment, while blood tests and subjective muscle soreness were assessed throughout the program. When all was said and done, the man who received the actual photobiomodulation therapy was lifting more, reported less fatigue, and had fewer blood biomarkers associated with inflammation.

Now, you might observe that a two-person study is awfully small. And that's true. But here's the kicker: The participants were 19-year-old twins who, in addition to being virtually genetically identical, were both college soccer players who lived together, trained together, and had the same dietary habits! And while it's true that even in twins, there can be many small differences that can impact a study's results, in this blind and placebo-controlled study, the only major difference was that one twin was unknowingly exposed to infrared light therapy and the other wasn't.[30]

Sexual Health

Up until just a few years ago, the people who were most likely to have heard of any sort of light therapy were probably those who knew about it in a dermatological context.

And then Tucker Carlson came along.

The veteran television host—who was at the time the most popular host on Fox News—had long been known as an ultra-conservative firebrand. But Carlson wasn't really known as someone with any interest, let alone expertise, in health and wellness. So, it was a bit surprising when Carlson decided to host an entire special about a "crash" in testosterone levels among American men, including a segment on what he termed "testicle tanning."

Perhaps less surprisingly, that term was trending on various social media sites within minutes.

If you missed all this back in the spring of 2022, we suspect you might have some questions. We're going to get to that soon. First, though, we need to talk about those purportedly falling testosterone levels: It's true—although not likely for the "lack of manliness" that Carlson and his guests were suggesting throughout the program. Like all hormones, testosterone tends to stay in balance when the rest of our health is in balance. As recent decades have brought a decline in health for Americans in general—owing to poor diets, bad exercise habits, increased weight, alcohol overuse, and terrible sleep—it's not at all surprising that a 2021 study of about 4,000 men found a roughly 25 percent decrease in serum testosterone levels among adolescent and young adult men between 1999 and 2016.[31]

The question about what to do about this problem is another matter altogether. And while Carlson was mocked for bringing it up (albeit almost exclusively by people on the opposite side of the political spectrum), he saw the humor, too. "So, obviously, half the viewers right now are like, 'What? Testicle tanning? That's crazy!'" Carlson said.

So why even bring it up? Because, as Carlson said, "Testosterone levels have crashed and nobody says anything about it. That's crazy. So why is it crazy to seek solutions?"

It's not. No matter how you might feel about Carlson's politics, the fact is that this is a problem that affects millions of people across the United

States and hundreds of millions around the world. And every day Restore staffers hear from people who are dealing with a lack of libido or another symptom of sexual dysfunction—and no one should ever be derided for asking questions about their own wellness.

Now, the reality is that there isn't any scientific evidence that suggests light therapy directly targeted on a man's testicles is an effective way to raise testosterone. But when we broaden the question to whether photobiomodulation can help with sexual health in general, a much clearer picture emerges. In studies of various forms of light therapy, photobiomodulation has been shown to impact the metabolism, motility, and viability of sperm as an apparent effect of its impact on mitochondria and ATP production.[32] It has also been shown to have a beneficial impact on sexual interest, sexual arousal, and orgasm in both men and women. In one case study from researchers at Massachusetts General Hospital, one patient "joked that he had been more sexually active with his girlfriend to the point that she had asked him to return to his own apartment and spend the following nights there." Upon experiencing a profound change in her libido, another patient in that same study told researchers that she was "perplexed" that photobiomodulation was not a popular intervention "and she equated her sexual functioning to her adolescence."[33]

The lesson here is that while light (like all the elements we've discussed in this book) isn't a panacea—and people do sometimes have strange ideas about how to apply it—it's also not something to deride just because it doesn't fit into mainstream views of how to promote better health. In hindsight, after all, everything we know about mainstream medical practices that are highly effective seems to make perfect sense. But if we didn't know that it works, what would we think if someone told us that tree bark can cure headaches? Well, that's where we got aspirin. What might we think about the idea of purposely injecting people with one virus to prevent another? That's the smallpox vaccine.

Not every crazy-sounding idea is a pathway to wellness. But any idea can be a pathway to personal investigation and—preferably guided by a physician whose views on wellness align with your own—exploration. And that's what we believe many people can and should be doing when it comes to light.

Not every crazy-sounding idea is a pathway to wellness. But any idea can be a pathway to personal investigation and—preferably guided by a physician whose views on wellness align with your own—exploration.

The Most Powerful Tailwind

We're big believers in the power of red light therapy. But if you're ready to realign your own circadian rhythms, a visit to one of our studios isn't necessarily the right place to start.

Instead, we suggest that you choose a day or two of living life in alignment with the sun—a 24- or 48-hour period in which you spend as much of your day as possible in natural light and as much of your night as possible with true darkness. That's what University of Colorado integrative physiologist Ken Wright advocates. For years, Wright has been leading camping trips in the Cache la Poudre Wilderness and other awe-inspiring locations across the Centennial State as demonstrations of his compelling hypothesis that just a few days lived in harmony with the spinning of Earth can restore balance in our lives.

In 2013, Wright sent volunteers on a camping trip in which they were exposed to four times more daylight, on average, than they got in their normal day-to-day lives, while being prohibited from using any form of unnatural light after the sun set. Before and afterward, the campers' levels of melatonin were tested, and those tests demonstrated a striking realignment in which their levels of that sleep-inducing hormone synced with the summer sun.[34] Similar studies conducted over the next few years confirmed that "the camping trick" works in both summer and winter, and in as little as two days.

This is good news if you like camping. But you don't have to head out into the great beyond to do this. All you must do is set your alarm clock to sunrise, spend as much time during the day outside your home or office, and pledge to avoid screens or electric lights after the sun sets. This takes planning and resolve. But it's a practice that most people could—and we believe should—work into their lives every now and then.

Few of us can do this more than occasionally, though. So, supplemental light—guided by research on the wavelengths that make the most sense for the wellness challenges you are targeting—can be an effective way to maintain our connection to this powerful element of hyper wellness. This is particularly true when light is stacked upon other therapies.

That's what Nathan, a retired elementary school principal from Jefferson County, Alabama, has discovered. "For me, red light feels like a force multiplier," he said. "I do regular cryotherapy. It makes me feel good. It gets me going for a day, and that's something that, if I take action with exercise and other things like that, I can keep going for a few days. But there's something about the red light therapy that accentuates those benefits. It keeps that flame going for a lot longer for me."

"For me, red light feels like a force multiplier."

We've heard similar stories from too many people to count. The reason is almost certainly that humans, like all animals that live on the surface of this planet, are deeply connected to the cycles of light in which we've evolved to live. And once we're reconnected to those rhythms, it's much easier for the next push we get—by way of any of the other elements—to keep us there.

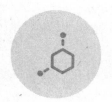

chapter 9

nourishment

As a college soccer player in the 1990s, Gina had been told by her coaches and trainers that it was important to keep her fat intake low, and she attempted to do that for many years as she tried to fight back against the weight gain that almost everyone experiences in their 20s. Then, in the early 2000s, she learned about the Atkins diet, which made her rethink her long avoidance of fat, and instead, she focused on shunning carbohydrates. And then, in the late 2010s, she learned about intermittent fasting, and began avoiding breakfast and lunch on most days to reduce her overall calories and trigger the healthy cellular stress responses that come from hunger.

"In between I tried all sorts of things that I heard would be good for me, and to be honest I don't know if any of these things has ever really helped," the 51-year-old park ranger from Bozeman, Montana, said. "Some things led to a little bit of weight loss for a short time, but after a year or two of doing something, I'd still step on the scale and see that I was a little heavier than when I started, and I'd start looking for something else that would be more effective."

All "good" diets share a few commonalities. They are made up of whole foods. They treat food as fuel. They limit overconsumption. And these principles could be embedded into any of the diets that Gina tried.

But none of those diets were specifically *designed* for any one person. Our genes are different. Our epigenomes are different. Our jobs, lifestyles, attitudes, vices, and exercise habits are different. So, while there are many ways of eating that can promote better health, in order to move toward hyper wellness it's important to move toward a better understanding of one's own uniqueness.

That's what Gina did, albeit nearly by accident. In the spring of 2022, a fellow veteran park ranger convinced Gina to join him at a Restore studio, where he was going to have a micronutrient biomarker assessment done. These assessments offer a snapshot of the levels of antioxidants, amino acids, and other micronutrients in a person's body, allowing clients to home in on insufficiencies and make informed decisions about their health.

"He had just gotten his genome done, and this was like step two for him. He was pretty excited about all this information he had and was hungry to get more," Gina explained. "Even though he was really enthusiastic, I wasn't convinced, but I was curious, and I've never been afraid of information, so I came along."

When Gina received her report, she realized something that had never occurred to her before. "I was reading the names of these substances that are in my body, and there were a lot of them that I didn't even know. But I had this moment when I recognized that what I was really looking at was an individualized picture of someone who was different from anyone else in the world. And it hit me that I had always been doing these diets that were marketed as if they were good for everyone. But I'm not everyone. I'm me."

Increasingly, people around the world are similarly rejecting one-size-fits-all dieting advice as they recognize that everyone has different nutritional needs that are driven by the differences in our genes, the expression of those genes, our lifestyles, our states of aging, and myriad other factors. Understanding how all those factors interact to create a surplus or deficiency of any one essential nutrient can be a tremendous challenge, and even an impossible one. But, thankfully, getting a much clearer picture of what nutrients are stable and healthy in your body, and which ones you might need more of, is relatively easy. All it takes is a test like the one Gina and her friend had done.

"I had always been doing these diets that were marketed as if they were good for everyone. But I'm not everyone. I'm me."

We hasten to note that micronutrient testing isn't proprietary to Restore. There are other reputable establishments offering similar testing, including through tests you can do at home. Doctors can also order these assessments for patients—although in many cases the costs to do these tests "in system" is much higher than it is to have them done privately, so exploration of all options can be beneficial.

After spending a bit of time on the internet investigating how to mitigate her reported deficiencies in potassium, leucine, vitamin C, and vitamin B12, Gina quickly recognized that she might benefit from eating more fruit. "I eat a lot of veggies. That's always been a constant in every diet I've tried. Fruit wasn't a priority, I guess because I was sort of suspicious of the sugars," she said. "So, I went to the store and got some apples and bananas, and I also got a little package of guavas, which I used to pick in my aunt's backyard when I was growing up in California, and I just told myself that I was going to add some fruit like this to my diet for a while and take a test again in a few months just to see what happened."

What happened, though, was that Gina recognized a palpable change in the way she felt long before she got her follow-up biomarker test. "I thought at first it was just the nostalgia of eating a guava, because my mood just brightened in those next few days and that was the only thing that made sense to me," she said.

We don't discount the power of nostalgia, but what Gina experienced when she increased her fruit consumption is also backed by multiple studies, including one in which researchers reviewed the food diaries of more than 12,000 people enrolled in one of Australia's largest long-term studies of eating habits. That study showed that the motivation to eat healthy food is weakened by the fact that most people believe the benefits only accrue years or decades down the line—and thus ostensibly cannot be seen or felt in the immediate moment. But if you ask people to focus on how they actually feel when they eat these foods, they are indeed able to identify immediate improvements in feelings of well-being and happiness.[1]

There's an important lesson here, and it's not just that an increased intake of fruits and veggies is good for most people—which, of course, is one of the oldest pieces of health advice given by doctors all over the world. Rather, what Gina experienced as she began making eating decisions based on her personal data was that the right-away impact became tangible.

"Eating for the now" makes a tremendous amount of sense when we consider what happens in the human body upon the consumption of any kind of food. Take an apple, for instance. Most of the nutrients will be completely transformed within an hour of having eaten that piece of fruit. In two hours, the converted molecules will have been dispersed into every system of the body, providing power for our cells. In three hours, that boost of energy will cap. In six hours, all but the residual molecular traces of the apple will be gone. In eight hours, even the remaining fibers in the gut will begin to leave the body.

Does eating a single apple have a long-term impact on one's health? Only in ways so minute that they could never even be measured. But that same piece of fruit has a tremendous impact on what happens in the immediate hours after it's first consumed. When Gina began to consider nutrition in this way—when she *nourished* her next moment rather than trying to guess at how today's decisions would impact her months, years, or decades into the future—she made much better choices.

"The feedback I was getting from my body became more noticeable," she said. "I think that was because I was actually looking for the effects of my food choices in the place and time that those effects actually occur, which is almost immediately after I eat, instead of trying to understand the effects in the long term, through weight loss."

And with that, just as is the case with the other elements of hyper wellness, the virtuous cycle has begun. For Gina, that meant more energy to exercise, which led her to resume playing soccer with a team of friends, which in turn sparked a competitive impulse that led her to work even harder to stay fit.

"I've been a bit of an evangelist for this way of thinking about nutrition, which cracks me up because the way I got started on this whole journey was through my friend, who I thought was being a bit of a zealot about his health data," she said. "But now just about everybody on my team shares a belief in eating in this way."

So, nourishment isn't just about what we eat. It's about how we eat. It's about how we supplement when food alone doesn't provide us with what our bodies need to function at a maximum level. And it's about tracking and adjusting over time as we experience aging and our needs change.

Food

At 35 years old, Meili was 75 pounds heavier than she had been when she graduated from college. "All that extra weight was getting in the way of the other things I wanted to do to improve my health," she said. "I could look at myself in a logical way and recognize that I was obese. But I tried a bunch of different diets. I couldn't stick to any of them. I was always cheating and always failing. It's honestly embarrassing."

Meili shouldn't have been embarrassed. Because while we often think about these sorts of challenges as something that can be overcome with just a little more willpower, the truth is that we aren't *just* in a battle with our wills, but with our very evolutionary programming.

Take sugar, for instance. People who live in the United States consume more than 300 percent of the recommended daily amount of added sugar, and this is one of the biggest factors in many people's weight gain.[2] But it's not just the fact that added sugar is so ubiquitous in processed foods that makes it difficult to stop consuming. It's also the fact that for our ancestors, a short-term burst of energy, particularly in the form of natural sugars, could be the difference between life and death. As such, the predecessors who evolved to perceive sugars as sweet, and to process sweetness as something desirable, had an advantage over their rivals. So too did those whose bodies best processed carbohydrates as sugars. Those are powerful selective forces!

In the sorts of timelines that drove our development as a species, the long-term individual consequences didn't matter much: From the standpoint of evolutionary survival, after all, what really mattered was being fit enough to become a parent and give offspring the protection they needed so that they would be likely to survive and be able to do the same. In the times of our most ancient human ancestors, that full cycle would have been 20 to 30 years, which happens to be how long our Stone Age ancestors are thought to have lived on average. Thus, the short-term benefits of sugar consumption were vast, while the long-term detriments were virtually inconsequential— up until relatively recently, that is, when far more of us began living well into our 60s and 70s and 80s. Meanwhile, food manufacturers learned that they could cheaply tap into our innate desire for foods that provide fast energy by hyper-charging those foods with heavily processed sugars.

With that, an epidemic was born. Today, around the world, 1 in 5 people over the age of 65 has type 2 diabetes, and it's projected that this share of the population will skyrocket in the next two decades as lifespans continue to increase and sugar- and carb-loaded foods become increasingly available globally.[3]

There are entire books written on the myriad other problems with modern diets. (Jason Fung's *The Obesity Code* and Michael Pollan's *Food Rules* are both great resources for a deep dive into how to eat for wellness in a world that has been designed for quick calories and constant satiation.) But the sugar-seeker's dilemma is a good example of why healthy eating practices aren't just a matter of "sticking to a diet." That's because the ways in which most people diet trigger biochemical changes that impact their neurological circuitry, hormonal balances, and metabolic processes[4]—even more evolutionary programming designed to make us want food when it's close at hand. And in the modern world, food is indeed almost always close at hand!

That's a problem that Meili could do something about in just one afternoon. In a matter of a few hours, she stripped her pantry bare of everything that had processed sugar in it, then went to the store to purchase only fruits, vegetables, whole grains, nuts, beans, nonprocessed meats, and milk. "At the very least, I wanted to make my home a place where the easiest thing to eat was going to be healthy for me," she told us in late 2022. "I knew I'd also need to control the way I was eating outside my house, because I eat a lot at restaurants, but I thought this would be a good first step."

This is not a step we would recommend for everyone. It was an extreme action that Meili took with the intention of making a sudden and substantial shift in how she eats, more akin to the idea of a "diet coup" that, as we noted earlier in this book, isn't generally the best way to make changes in our relationship to nourishment. For Meili, though, it worked. Having whole foods close at hand helped her feel more satiated and more energetic—two right-away benefits that she was able to leverage toward other healthy actions, including more exercise and hot-cold contrast therapy. When we last checked in with her, she'd been on the virtuous cycle for about a year and had dropped 20 pounds.

But no matter what foods you are putting into your body, and no matter how healthy those foods may be, it's important to consider ways in which you might be able to eat less, eat less often, or both. This is a step beyond limiting overconsumption; it's work toward understanding and pursuing the minimal amount of consumption necessary that still provides adequate nutrition.

One of the most compelling ongoing studies of the benefits of eating less—caloric restriction—is happening at Duke University, where the Comprehensive Assessment of Long-Term Effects of Reducing Intake of Energy (yes, the homophonic acronym is CALERIE) has been ongoing since the early 2000s, producing dozens of research findings. In one phase of the project, the researchers conducted a randomized controlled trial involving more than 200 people, half of whom were given information and support for a diet that would restrict their caloric intake by 25 percent over a period of two years. The participants didn't reach that goal—the average reduction was about 12 percent—but they nonetheless became a tremendous example for why any step in the right direction is a tailwind to celebrate, for they experienced profound health improvements over the control group, with lower blood pressure, lower cholesterol, lower rates of diabetes, lower risk factors for heart disease and stroke, and lower levels of inflammation.[5]

Another increasingly popular pathway toward potentially similar results, even without reducing calories overall, is time-restricted eating—keeping all meals to a set period of the day and leaving plenty of time in between for your body to fully metabolize the fuel you have provided for it. This is a more controversial approach, with mixed results in a variety of settings, but when a team of Korean researchers analyzed data from 19 studies that were conducted around the world, they found that people who are able to condense healthy eating patterns into fewer hours of the day experienced weight loss, fat loss, lowered blood pressure, lowered blood glucose, and healthier cholesterol levels.[6]

In the same way that people who stage a "diet coup" often end up abandoning that approach, caloric restriction and time-restricted eating are unlikely to work if done all at once. Remember: It's easier to build capacity by building on the tailwinds you already have. Reducing portion sizes, even by a small amount, is a form of caloric restriction. Taking breakfast a half-hour later than normal is a start toward time-restricted eating.

Food isn't the only answer to the challenge of nourishment, but it really should be the primary answer. We evolved to get most of our nutrients from food, so we should indeed get most of our nutrients from food. And yes, we can be assured that this will provide vast health advantages many years down the road. But we should also look for and enjoy the benefits that healthy foods offer us *right away*.

Food isn't the only answer to the challenge of nourishment, but it really should be the primary answer.

In most cases, though, even those who understand this principle and eat in exceptionally healthy ways will begin to experience temporary and chronic nutrient deficiencies as they age, resulting in a vicious cycle that can accentuate aging, thus further promoting nutrient insufficiencies. Thus, once we're moving toward hyper wellness in the ways in which we approach food, it also becomes helpful to begin thinking about supplementation.

Supplementation

Despite a lifelong history of asthma and a more recent diagnosis of ulcerative colitis, Christopher had always led an active life. The Dallas native loved to travel, mountain bike, hike, and garden, and since the medications he was on seemed to be working, he had every intention of doing those things for many decades to come.

But as Christopher got closer and closer to his 40th birthday, it was clear that something wasn't right. "I just kept ratcheting up my medications, and they were less and less effective," he said. "The first thing that had to go was travel, because with an inflammatory bowel condition, long trips were more risky, but it wasn't long before I really wasn't able to get very far from my home or office at all, so the outdoors things I was doing were out because, you know, I have to be close to a bathroom. And then on top of that, it was taking all my energy just to get through the workday, and I was so winded and tired that even going into the backyard was really hard."

As the vice president for technology at a midsized bank, Christopher felt fortunate to have good health care coverage, but he was unsatisfied by what his doctors were telling him about his situation. "Basically it was 'Just keep increasing the drugs' and 'This will just continue to get worse and worse as time goes by,' and there was just no talk of recovery and no hope whatsoever," he said. "It was devastating."

Discontented with the conventional answers he was getting, Christopher found a homeopathic holistic doctor who was willing to take a different approach. "And he said, 'Look, your body is out of balance, so first we need to figure out the ways in which you're imbalanced and then make some decisions about what to do about that.' And that's how I wound up at Restore," he said, "because my doctor said we should start fresh with doing some new bloodwork and it was actually cheaper and faster to do it there."

The first thing that Christopher noticed when he got his first micronutrient biomarker report in June 2022 was how easy it was to read. A typical comprehensive metabolic panel report includes a measurement of 14 different substances in a person's blood along with reference ranges, all reported as numbers. The report he got from Restore included dozens of biomarkers each reported on a color-coded scale—green for sufficient, yellow for borderline, and red for insufficient.

"And man, there was a lot of red and yellow on that thing," Christopher recalled.

The report showed that Christopher was deeply deficient in biotin, ar-
ginine, manganese, strontium, and glutathione. He was also borderline
for vitamin K2, vitamin B3, chromium, copper, molybdenum, selenium,
asparagine, and tyrosine. "And even the stuff that was in the green was
right on the edge of the borderline range," he said. "There wasn't much
that seemed to be really good."

In consultation with his doctor, Christopher returned to the Restore
studio to receive an IV drip specifically aimed at the nutrients his body
was most deficient in. "The thing I shake my head at now is that this actually seems like the simplest and most straightforward thing to do, right?
Like, you see what's missing and you try to replace it. That makes so much
sense," he said. "But that wasn't something any of my other doctors had
even suggested. It was just more drugs, more drugs, more drugs."

As he was driving home from his first IV drip appointment, Christopher said, he felt a rush of energy. "Maybe it was just the thought that I
was doing something new," he said, "but I still felt better the next day, and
that's a really big motivator to just keep doing it."

Every week he got a drip. And every week he felt a little better. His
energy was returning. As a result, he was exercising more. And true to the
power of the virtuous cycle, that exercise led to some weight loss, which
led Christopher to feel better about himself, which led him to take steps
to improve his diet as well. That step might have been one of the reasons
that he was having fewer painful ulcerative colitis flare-ups. He was also
breathing better, so he began weaning himself off the higher level of medications he had been taking. He returned to the garden. He started hiking
again. He got back on his mountain bike. And, when we last spoke with
him, he and his husband were planning a trip to Europe. "In pretty much
every way, my life was transformed," he said.

Six months after starting IV therapy, Christopher followed up with
another biomarker test, which showed vast improvements in almost every
nutrient he'd been deficient or borderline on in the first assessment. "So,

in that first report, I had five red marks and eight yellow," he said. "And six months later there were just two things in the red and three in yellow, and that was totally affirming, but I have to say that I didn't even need that report to tell me what I already knew. My life had been changed so much."

"In pretty much every way, my life was transformed."

Around that same time, Christopher had a colonoscopy, a common test for people with ulcerative colitis. "And my colorectal surgeon told me everything looked better than ever," he said. "He was also impressed that my cholesterol was way lower and my blood pressure was lower, too, especially when I told him I had stopped taking a lot of the meds I was on before. So, he asked me what I was doing, and I told him, but he really didn't seem to believe it."

If Christopher hadn't lived through such a profoundly transformational experience, he wouldn't have believed it either. "I'm a tech guy," he said. "For me, the bottom line is always data, and my data is so obvious."

Earlier in this book, we noted that much of the immediate power of IV drips comes from the simple fact that almost everyone feels better when they're better hydrated, but there's a growing body of evidence that IV supplementation of nutrients can have an impact far beyond hydration.

Magnesium, for instance, has been copiously studied in patients with asthma, and a meta-analysis of ten separate trials demonstrated that IV magnesium sulfate treatment is associated with significant effects on respiratory function and a reduction in hospitalization.[7] Intravenous glutathione, which is found in plants and animals and is a well-studied antioxidant, has also been evaluated for its potential to reduce damage to a person's heart cells after a major heart attack, with one randomized control trial showing that, compared to a placebo, glutathione was effective at improving the survival of cardiomyocytes.[8]

We always want to be transparent about what the research does and doesn't demonstrate, and in the case of IV therapy there have certainly been studies that have suggested either a weak or nonexistent effect, including one study that indicated that IV magnesium isn't a good way to address muscle cramps,[9] another that put a damper on hopes that IV magnesium would help reduce mortality after a stroke,[10] and yet another that showed that an IV including the trace mineral selenium didn't improve short-term survival in a group of patients who suffered from acute respiratory distress syndrome, an accumulation of fluid in the lungs that sometimes occurs as the result of a bad infection, especially in older patients with other underlying health conditions.[11]

What you may have noticed, though, is that all these studies—both those with positive results and those where the evidence of benefit was lacking—were conducted on patients with significant or severe health conditions. Alas, like most of the research that backs the other therapies we've discussed in this book, much of the research into IV supplementation has been conducted on unhealthy people.

Not all of it, though. For instance, intravenous vitamin C has demonstrated promising results when it comes to reducing markers for inflammation[12] and fatigue[13] in generally healthy test subjects. Can we surmise from these findings that IV administration of other nutrients will also be effective in healthy subjects? Not really. And that's why many people like Robert Shmerling, the former clinical chief of the division of rheumatology at Boston's Beth Israel Deaconess Medical Center, have expressed hesitation about IV supplementation, even though, as Shmerling conceded in 2018, "the medical risks are low."

"Keep in mind that the fluids and other therapies offered can be readily obtained in other ways, (drinking fluids, taking generic vitamins, and other over-the-counter medications) for only a few bucks," Shmerling wrote.[14]

But we'll take that one step further. Why on Earth would you take generic vitamins and over-the-counter medications—the latter of which *always* come with a risk of side effects—if you can simply let food be your medicine? If you are like Gina or Meili, and find that you can step onto the virtuous cycle with a shift in food-based nourishment, why wouldn't you start there? It would be foolish not to.

Why on Earth would you take generic vitamins and over-the-counter medications—the latter of which always *come with a risk of side effects—if you can simply let food be your medicine?*

At this point, though, we've lost track of the number of people who have told us that they were either trying their best to follow doctor-prescribed dietary advice or, like Christopher, were so overwhelmed by chronic illnesses that a dramatic shift in diet felt impossible without some other sort of boost. That's why if you walk into any Restore studio in the nation, at virtually any time of the day, you'll find people from all walks of life lounging together in the drip therapy room, IVs in arm, often chatting about their lives and the events that led them to this therapy.

On one recent day in Salt Lake City, for instance, there was Ignacio, who had first come into a Restore for an IV drip several years earlier when he was working for a company that laid fiber optic cables across the largely desert state of Utah. "We'd work outside all day and I got so dehydrated that my boss got worried and he drove me straight here," he said. "But a few years ago I quit that job and opened my own restaurant, and then we were successful so I opened another. I no longer get dehydrated, but I have a lot of stress and need a lot of energy, because it's not so physical anymore but it's mentally taxing and I always feel very drained."

Next to Ignacio was Laurie, a professional singer who had flown in from New Orleans with some girlfriends for a ski trip in nearby Park City. She had started using IV therapy after a bout with long COVID in 2020, "and it worked so well for me that it turned into a regular routine."

And across from Laurie sat Erin, who had recently had a baby—nearly 20 years after she had given birth to her first child. "It's a lot harder this time," she laughed. "I feel more tired and more drained, but I want to be just as good of a mother for my new son as I was for my two other children even though I might be a lot older now."

In the roughly 30 minutes that their appointments overlapped, Laurie and Erin commiserated on their shared experiences with long COVID. Erin got the address to Ignacio's restaurant and promised that she would visit soon. And Ignacio told Laurie about his favorite restaurants in Park City. And we sat back and reveled in what we were hearing: Not just the stories of three people who have found this therapy to be effective in their own lives, but a conversation between three strangers who built a connection with one another.

IM Shots

Not everyone is so chatty and extroverted as Laurie, Erin, and Ignacio were on the day we met them in Utah. And not everyone who feels they need the benefits of an IV drip always has the time it takes to complete that therapy, which can take 60 to 90 minutes.

That's why we've become big fans of intramuscular shots, which are a faster way to get many of the same nutrients into your body, and a quickly growing therapy especially among competitive athletes.

That includes Keon, a track and field athlete who trains in several states during the year and who, as a vegan, is more vulnerable to being deficient in vitamin B12. This vitamin, which is prevalent in dairy products, eggs, fish, meat, and poultry, is essential to maintain brain function, promote healthy blood and nerve cells, and make DNA. IM shots are also permitted in moderation for college and professional athletes, and thus a common way to restore energy.

"I wouldn't mind taking a break in the middle of the day to get an IV drip of B12, but an hour or more really is out of the question for me," Keon told us. "The shots take ten minutes or less. And within a few hours I feel amazing. Both my body and my mind feel sharper and stronger."

B12 shots aren't a closely held secret, or really any sort of secret at all. One study of track and field athletes in Europe concluded that more than a third of the competitors were using B12 injections, and among endurance athletes specifically an even greater percentage were using B12 shots.[15]

"The shots take ten minutes or less. And within a few hours I feel amazing. Both my body and my mind feel sharper and stronger."

Another popular intramuscular shot is vitamin D, which many people recognize as the vitamin we get from the sun. What many people don't know is that there is a specific receptor for vitamin D on almost every cell in the human immune system, and that copious scientific studies have affirmed that this nutrient plays an outsize role in healthy immune function.[16] Put simply: Vitamin D helps us beat infections of all sorts. Yet we spend far less time in the sun than our ancestors and, as a possible result, more than a third of the population of the United States is deficient in this essential vitamin.[17] Researchers in India have demonstrated that oral supplementation and intramuscular shots are both effective ways to raise vitamin D. That study found that the levels dropped after six weeks for those who took an oral supplement once per week for six weeks. In those who received just one injection, the levels of vitamin D continued to grow for at least twelve weeks after administration![18] Meanwhile, a small study of adults between the ages of 35 and 91 in Australia indicated that an intramuscular injection was safe and effective at raising and sustaining levels of vitamin D for a 24-week period,[19] and that same timeframe was backed by a similar and larger study of Korean adults between the ages of 19 and 65.[20]

Another common intramuscular shot is glutathione, which has been called the "master antioxidant" for its role in detoxification, antiviral defense, and immune response.[21] It is being investigated for its benefits in slowing and reversing skin aging,[22] improving COVID-19 recovery,[23] and mitigating neurological diseases such as Huntington's, Parkinson's, Alzheimer's, and stroke.[24] Much of this research is nascent, and there are many questions left to answer about this molecule, but it's nonetheless a popular supplement as both an IV ingredient and injection.

For many people, IVs and injections like those that are provided at Restore studios are simply not in the cards. But like nearly every other therapy in this book, there are alternatives. And in this case that alternative is the very thing that most people think of first when they think of "supplements."

Oral supplements can be effective, but it's important to note that these are products that are essentially sold and regulated as food ingredients—they aren't regulated for effectiveness and are often inaccurately labeled,[25] making third-party purity testing from reputable organizations like NSF (formerly the National Sanitation Foundation) vitally important. None of this is to say, however, that oral supplements don't work—they most certainly do for many people and many conditions. Indeed, surveys have suggested that a vast majority of doctors and nurses use dietary supplements themselves.[26]

If you do choose to bolster your nutrient intake through oral supplements, IV drips, or shots, what's right for you? Literally, the answer is "something that's completely different from what's right for anyone else in the world."

That might sound like an impossible puzzle to solve. And we won't lie to you: It can be difficult. But remember that building capacity isn't about getting the right answer. It's about identifying just one thing that makes you feel better right away.

Filling Your Sail

It's obviously important to think about your long-term future. And it can be a powerful exercise, too: Researchers have found that when people visualize their future self—and commit to caring for that person—they can better employ the self-control it takes to make healthy decisions in the present.[27]

But whether you are choosing a meal, taking an oral supplement, receiving an IV drip, or getting an intramuscular shot, a vital but all-too-often completely ignored question is: "What will this do for me right away?"

When nourishment of any sort supports an immediate boost in wellness of the mind and body, it generates capacity, which we are confident you now recognize as the currency that permits us to dedicate more energy to even more healthful actions. It permits for better and more prolonged exercise, for deeper sleep, and for building stronger connections with those who are important to us. Nourishment even begets more nourishment.

Few of us have been socialized to think about nutrition in this way, so it's important to apply some mindfulness to the moments and hours that follow any sort of nourishment. Be attentive to immediate signals. Do you feel sharper in body and mind? Did you notice a boost in energy? Most vitally to the virtuous cycle, did it help you do something else to promote greater wellness? If so, you're one step closer to finding the pattern of nourishment that's right for you. And, yes, that pattern might end up looking something like one of the diets that have been widely promoted and successfully utilized for greater health. But chances are good that it simply won't look that way. Because, as Gina noted, you're not everyone else. You're you.

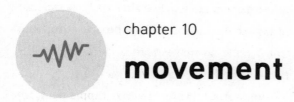

chapter 10

movement

After gaining nearly 20 pounds during the first year of the COVID-19 pandemic, Sergei looked at himself in the mirror one morning and decided he didn't at all like what he was seeing. Then and there, he committed to getting into better shape. "I went right to my closet, pulled out my old pair of running shoes, went to the local high school, and started running around the track," the psychiatrist said. "I knew I'd be sore, but that night my back was so tight that I couldn't even get out of bed. It was like that for three weeks."

It almost goes without saying that exercise is an essential component of wellness, but the vast majority of people who begin an exercise regimen in the two most common ways—running and going to the gym—quit within a few months, often because, just like Sergei, one or more injuries leave them less well than they were when they started. And yet many people who start and stop and start and stop an exercise routine keep going back to the same thing that didn't work in the first place. That's clearly a recipe for failure.

A physical therapist who worked just down the road from Sergei's office on Mesa Street in El Paso, Texas, was able to help Sergei get on better footing—starting with a regimen of nothing more than stretching. "That's all I was doing. Even when my back was feeling better she told me that she didn't want me to do anything else," Sergei said. "She just wanted me to go through this long routine of stretches."

It was a month before the physical therapist added anything else to the routine, but once again it was nothing particularly exertive. Now, she told Sergei, he needed to integrate some balancing exercises into the stretching regimen.

After another month of this, Sergei was beginning to feel frustrated. "I listened to her, because I know what it's like to offer a patient a pathway intended to help them and to have them ignore it," he said. "But none of this stuff was helping me lose weight, and I felt like all that motivation I'd had months earlier was dissipating."

Next, the therapist began leading Sergei through a series of weight training exercises—with what Sergei perceived to be embarrassingly small weights. "I kept reminding her that my goal was weight loss, and she assured me we'd get there, but I was doing the calculations in my head," he said. "If I'd been running all that time I'd be burning so many calories each day, and if I kept it up each day, that's times seven, and then multiply that by all those weeks that I was just doing these little exercises that weren't helping me reach that goal."

More than three months into their work together, the physical therapist finally cleared Sergei to run. "But only on two conditions," she told him. "First, you have to keep doing all these other exercises, and second, you need a recovery routine."

Sergei agreed, and his physical therapist laid out several options for post-exercise recovery. Together they settled on sauna because there were several places near his office he could go for that. "Every day after work I shut my door and do my stretches and other exercises, and then three days a week I go for a run and then finish at the sauna," Sergei explained.

Almost immediately, Sergei said, he felt like a fool for ever having doubted his physical therapist. "It was a completely different experience from what had happened when I just decided to go start running again on a whim," he said. "It was like my body was primed. And my recovery routine seemed to really be working to keep me from getting so sore and achy that I'd ever even think about taking a day off." Much to the contrary, in fact, he started adding even longer runs on the weekends.

"It was like my body was primed."

Over the next year, Sergei logged more than 600 miles of running—with no injuries—and he lost almost 20 pounds.

When Sergei's weight loss plateaued after about a year, he redirected his energy into a better diet, and began supplementing in areas where a biomarker report showed he was deficient. That resulted in more energy, which he put into more exercise. He now logs more than 1,000 miles of running a year and hasn't been injured since beginning this routine.

Many people might observe that the secret to Sergei's success is that, after facing that first obstacle, his physical therapist was able to convince him to "start slow." That's one way to look at it. What we saw was a man who had one gusty but not very sustainable tailwind—the motivation to get back to exercising to lose weight—and who instead was compelled by a smart therapist to build up other supportive tailwinds, little by little, investing greater flexibility into balance, investing balance into strength, and investing strength into endurance. Moreover, the therapist ensured that a huge headwind—the aches and pains that come with aging—was being mitigated through the use of sauna, a therapy that has been well studied for its impact on exercise recovery.[1]

Whether you're trying to get back to exercising or trying to maximize the benefits that you're already getting from a well-established exercise program, it's important to recognize that whenever you accentuate a tailwind or mitigate a headwind, little things really do matter.

That doesn't mean it's not possible to take *big* initial steps. We know plenty of people who have made a drastic shift in their exercise regimen and reaped amazing benefits as a result. But what the data tells us is that for most people, most of the time, the secrets to long-term success in this essential part of a healthy life are moderation, intentionality, and commitment.

Accentuating the Tailwinds of Movement

As we were mapping out the nine elements of hyper wellness, the choice to use the word "movement" instead of "exercise" was intentional, because while the trappings of our modern world make deliberate physical exertion imperative, our species didn't evolve to exercise in this purposeful and repetitious way. Rather, we evolved—like most other creatures—to be in a nearly constant state of movement simply as a condition of our life's circumstances. Climbing on trees and rocks. Swimming through lakes and trudging through streams. Running from predators. Playing with friends and family members. Foraging and hunting for food. It wasn't until the advent of agriculture, about 10,000 years ago in some societies and far more recently in others, that *repetitive* movement became such a big part of human lives. Even then, movement itself was nearly constant.

Movement is thus a tailwind reinforced by evolutionary momentum, and we can and should take advantage of that. It might seem commonsensical to start by identifying the parts of our life that are most sedentary and doing what we can to make them less so, but turning inertia into momentum takes a lot more energy than turning momentum into more momentum.

This is where another form of personal census comes into play: From the time you arise from your bed in the morning until the time you lie down again each night, what movement is *already* built into your life? Can those individual movements be accentuated to work toward greater balance, more flexibility, improved endurance, and greater strength?

By way of example, it takes a little bit of movement just to put on our clothes in the morning, but we generally rush through this part of our routine without recognizing it as an opportunity to more deliberately move through the process. Stretching an arm through a shirt sleeve. Standing on one leg and then the other to put on a pair of pants. Bending down to slip on a shoe. Slowing down by just a few seconds for each movement is a way to accentuate this tailwind of existing movement.

If you already walk from your front door to your car each morning, then you have an opportunity to raise your knees a little higher than is normal (and yes, a little higher than what will *look* normal to your neighbors). If you already park in a large lot at work, then parking a little farther away gives you an opportunity to take longer, stretching steps across the lot. If you already take the stairs at work (and of course you should), then taking two stairs at once or using the bottom step of each flight to get a deep calf flex is a good way to accentuate the movements you're already doing. If you use a wheelchair or other mobility assistance device, you're likely already exerting a lot of additional energy and time to getting from "here" to "there" thanks to cities and buildings that are all too often designed with accessibility as an afterthought—but you're also the absolute expert on what features of a street or building present challenges that you might choose to confront on your own volition to accentuate a tailwind.

To be clear: This isn't simply a way to "get started." This way of approaching movement throughout the day is something that anyone can take advantage of, no matter how healthy they might already be. In fact, if you're a person who is already doing a lot of *intentional* exercise, this might be one of the few places where you can draw a huge benefit.

Taking on the Headwinds of Motion

Once we've built some added action onto the movements we're already doing, it becomes valuable to start thinking about how we can convert inertia into momentum. That starts with identifying the most sedentary parts of our lives and doing what we can to make those periods of time less stationary.

The average American is sedentary for 9.5 hours of the time they are awake,[2] and whether you're far below or much above that mean, it's likely that you can easily identify some areas of your life in which your body isn't in motion. In fact, that might be the case at this very moment!

For most people, there are two major chunks of relative stillness—screen time and, in many professions, work time—and both generally offer some easy opportunities to convert inaction into movement.

In office settings, standing desks used to be unusual. These days there's hardly an office that doesn't have at least a few people who are working upright, and more and more of these folks aren't just standing but walking on treadmills. And whereas the person who was figuratively tied to their desk used to be the symbol of productivity, today many employers recognize that frequent breaks for movement improve worker efficiency and effectiveness.[3] Yet even if you've taken some or all these literal steps in your place of work, there's likely something else you could be doing to add more movement to your day. And, again, it's important to note that it doesn't have to be a big change to build capacity—even small things matter—and that goes for people who don't work at a desk, too. One extra flight of stairs instead of the elevator. One extra short break to walk around the block instead of sitting down in a break room. Walking or riding a bike instead of driving to work. Deliberate exercise during lunch. There's no one-size-fits-all prescription for movement, though, so we're not going to belabor this point. The important thing is to evaluate your own situation, recognize the opportunities to increase your movement, and then make it happen in a sustainable way.

Likewise, it was once common for people to return home after a hard day at work and immediately plop down on a chair or sofa to watch whatever happened to be on television. In fact, for many people, this was the image of a successful life. But even as the television has become a less central feature of many homes, screens have become an even bigger part of people's lives, and of course most of the time we are engaged in a screen we are moving little if at all. The good news is that pretty much everyone already knows how bad this is. We've met few people who don't understand that they spend far more time watching shows—and scrolling through social media—than they should.

The important thing is to evaluate your own situation, recognize the opportunities to increase your movement, and then make it happen in a sustainable way.

As the old adage goes, admitting you have a problem is the first step. What's the next step after that? Once again, while big changes—swearing off all unnecessary screen time and recommitting all those hours to movement—could make a huge difference in your life, you're far more likely to have greater success if you build upon a series of small changes. Turn social media into a reward for exercise. Commit to binge-watching TV shows only when you're on an exercise bike, treadmill, or rowing machine. Make a "no screens in the bedroom" pact with your partner (and then do other, more active, activities while in bed together!). We're not going to suggest there's a singular answer that works for everyone when it comes to movement, but absolutely everyone can turn their headwinds into tailwinds. Minute by minute, if need be, when you replace sedentary screentime with active motion, you are creating capacity that can be invested in more healthy activities.

The Right Motivation

A few years ago, we came upon an article called "The Best Workout Routine Ever, According to Science."

When it comes to the art and science of search engine optimization, that's a great title. Other than that, though, that headline was really a load of crap. There's no such thing as a "best workout," and no serious scientist would ever suggest so. And that includes Jeffrey Willardson, the "neuro-muscular adaptations to physical training" expert who devised the work-out in question—even he does not seem to have claimed that the workout was the "best" at anything.[4]

Willardson's workout comprises 10 exercises, 10 to 15 reps each, done consecutively with no rest in between, producing "fatigue but not failure." We know people who have tried it out, and it's been fantastic for some of them. But the "some" part of that equation is key, because what's right for you when it comes to intentional exercise is different from what's right for anyone else in the world.

So, for some people, something akin to Willardson's strength and conditioning routine will be just right. For others it's basketball, running, swimming, hiking, fencing, or something else! For most people, it's a combination of *many* different activities because, as has often been said, the best workout is one that a person will actually do. That's a generally good observation, but there's another important element, relative to the virtuous cycle: The best workout is one that provides an immediate, palpable feeling of wellness. If what you're doing to get exercise doesn't provide right-away positive feedback, then it isn't likely to be generating capacity for other actions, and it's going to be hard to sustain.

That's why we're huge proponents of experimentation—not only for those who are trying to get more intentional exercise into their lives but also for those who are lifelong athletes but don't feel an immediate sense of betterment every time they exercise. If you have been running for years, that's a good tailwind and you should absolutely keep going. But if you're not still making gains toward your full potential of healthfulness—and if your body is not increasingly capable of doing what it's designed to do with as little intervention as possible—then it's time to investigate other options. This doesn't mean replacing your running habit; there's a lot of good momentum there, after all. Rather, it might simply mean augmenting that activity with something else to explore how that supplemental activity makes you feel.

That's what Gus did. After retiring from the US Army, he tried to keep up the same regimen of exercises he'd done throughout his career in the Military Police Corps. "I was doing all the same stuff, but I wasn't getting the same benefit," he told us. "I could almost feel the weight of my age holding me down. My run times were slower. My max lifts were decreasing. I do understand that some of that comes with aging. But the downward trajectory was scary."

Everything changed for Gus when his granddaughter had a birthday party at a local ice rink. "I had played hockey as a kid, and when I got back on the ice, just skating around with those little kids, something just clicked," he said. "I started going back by myself, during the hours when the rink was pretty empty, just skating around, fooling around really, and I even took some lessons from a figure skating coach, which I never would have had the guts to do when I was younger."

Here's the important part: Every time Gus stepped off the ice, he felt better about himself. "I used to exercise to stay fit for my job, so there was a purpose that was driving me when I was running and lifting," he said. "When I retired, I think I lost that purpose. Then I started skating, and I had another purpose. Now, when I run and lift it's because I want to make sure I can keep skating for as long as possible."

We know people who worked their way through a seemingly endless list of activities—from running and swimming to biking and yoga, from Pilates to CrossFit, from team sports to pickleball—before coming upon the exercise regimen that met the "feel better" requirement. The hard truth is that finding what is right for you isn't always easy. It might be especially hard for people who have been exercising a certain way for a long time, without the "feel good" kick, because it's easier to just keep doing what they've been doing. But if what you're doing isn't still helping you make gains toward hyper wellness, then you're not treading water—you're losing ground—and exploration really is crucial.

If what you're doing isn't still helping you
make gains toward hyper wellness, then you're
not treading water—you're losing ground.

This is especially true because as we experience aging, we become more susceptible to injury. If you get exercise in only one way, and an injury prevents that exercise from continuing for a short time, the opportunity to get back to that activity might be a motivation. That's a potentially good thing. But if an injury prevents a return to that activity for a long time—or if an injury means "retirement" from that form of exercise—and you don't have something else to look forward to, you're in a real bind. Thus, the moment you arrive at something that works for you is not the moment to stop looking for other things; it's the exact right time to invest the energy you'll get from one "feel better" activity to finding another.

Thanks to its great weather, diverse and accepting culture, sports-obsessed atmosphere, and overall positive vibe, Austin has become a place where a lot of former professional athletes come to retire after leaving their careers in baseball, football, basketball, hockey, and soccer. But after living in this city for a long time, we've noticed that a lot of former pros, having spent decades dedicated to one specific sport, can have a difficult time staying fit once they're not training for that sport full-time—especially if injuries they suffered during their sports career have made certain types of exercise painful or impossible. This is a classic outcome of "identity foreclosure"—rigid commitment to a particular way of life or worldview—which is common among driven people when something central to their life is no longer present.[5] If that can happen to deeply motivated athletes who have spent a lifetime learning to maintain peak shape, it can happen to anyone who doesn't have more than one physical activity that brings them a sense of right-away well-being.

Vigorous Exercise

For those who are already engaged in regular, vigorous exercise, the principles we've been discussing so far in this chapter may be some of the best ways to squeeze a little more juice out of the orange, so to speak. We've yet to meet anyone, no matter how epically fit, who—upon thinking about opportunities to get a little more stretching, balancing, strengthening, and endurance exercise out of the things they're already doing—can't identify at least one part of their life in which they can accentuate a tailwind or mitigate a headwind to greater benefit.

For those who use these practices to get started on a fitness journey or to get back into better physical fitness after some time, though, here's a sometimes hard-to-hear truth: If the small steps you take to promote greater movement in your life don't ultimately lead to vigorous exercise, you will soon stall out in your progress toward hyper wellness.

When we say "vigorous exercise," what we mean are actions that require a high level of effort and result in an increase in your heart rate and respiration—activities that bring a dose of healthy stress to your life, triggering biochemical responses that have been shown to improve mitochondrial function,[6] reduce chronic inflammation,[7] improve insulin sensitivity,[8] and promote cardiovascular health.[9]

For most people who are in even halfway decent shape, this won't be accomplished with a jog, a leisurely bike ride, an easygoing swim, or a quick walk around the block. You've got to work for it, and the immediately positive, palpable feelings won't come without some physical discomfort first. A good rule of thumb is that if you can hold a conversation while exercising, you're probably not doing vigorous exercise.

As Sergei learned, it's not always wise to jump right into a vigorous exercise regimen if you've not already been through a few loops of capacity building via the virtuous cycle. And even once you have gained some momentum in this way, it's important to follow right-away successes with reasonable steps in the same direction.

If you can hold a conversation while exercising, you're probably not doing vigorous exercise.

That's what makes high-intensity interval training (HIIT) such a natural fit for many people who are initially pursuing a feel-better-do-more lifestyle. The individual exercises in a HIIT program can be as short as 10 seconds, and the reps, rest, and total session time can all be adjusted to individual abilities. A HIIT workout that includes just 10 to 20 seconds each of jumping jacks, squats, lunges, and running in place would be an accessible start for many people—a way to get one's heart beating and lungs burning. If that small dose results in a palpable feeling of betterment, then it's something that can be built upon, a few seconds or a few reps at a time.

HIIT isn't the right approach for everyone when it comes to vigorous exercise. The right approach, as we noted earlier, is to identify the exercises that you can and will actually do, that make you feel better right away, and that therefore create capacity for other steps toward hyper wellness. And because vigorous exercise does put greater strains on our bodies, particularly as we age, it's doubly important to diversify activities that do all these things, so that you have some options on the table if you're unable to engage in a primary regimen for any reason.

One of our clients in southern Louisiana, Roy, has been a remarkable example of how to safely and successfully integrate vigorous exercise into one's life. It had been years since the competitive club soccer coach had played the game he was teaching to young men and women in his community, and during that time he'd failed to add any other vigorous activities to his life.

"I'd stopped playing soccer when I was 27 or 28 because my ankles kept rolling on me," he said. "I always figured I was staying in decent shape because I wasn't gaining a ton of weight, and I was definitely getting exercise just being around the kids all the time, jogging around, passing the ball around, and all that, but I wasn't training or competing—not in soccer and not in anything else."

It was an invitation to play pickleball with his father that made Roy realize that he needed to get back to some sort of vigorous activity. "He's 30 years older than I am and he kicked my butt," Roy told us. "He kept saying that it was just because he knew how to play and I didn't, but that wasn't true. I was gasping for air and it was like my heart was beating out of my chest."

The explosion of interest in pickleball over the past few years has been a marvelous thing. The sport is designed to be able to be played by just about anyone, so even people who are not in the best of shape can easily get started—which is one of the things that has contributed to its popularity among older Americans. What you get out of the game is also what you put in—so if you want a round of pickleball to knock you on your butt, it will.

Roy started playing with his father every morning before work. "It was great for me, not just because I was getting exercise but because we were able to just spend some time together," he said. "And it was rough at first, but it's really a game you can play even if you're not huffing and puffing, but then work your way up to exercise that, for me at least, was making me feel the way I used to feel when I'd have a good, hard soccer practice."

The benefits helped him work more vigorously on the soccer field as a coach as well. "I was mixing it up with the kids a bit more than I did," he said. "And they noticed. One kid started calling me Coach Speedy, which I don't exactly love as a nickname, but I guess it's better than some alternatives."

Now that he's once again able to engage in vigorous exercise, Roy has also started swimming on the weekends. "I've managed to avoid hurting my ankles again, but I knock on wood every time I mention that," he said. "If it does happen, I know I'll still be able to swim, so I can stay in shape even while I'm recovering from that."

Recovery

There's another rule of thumb that can be a good guide to determining whether you are getting vigorous exercise, particularly if you haven't been doing much of it in the past: You really need to *feel it* the next day.

Roy was definitely feeling the effects of his new pickleball routine when we first met him at a Restore studio near New Orleans. Indeed, that's why he was there, getting ready to head into the sauna. "I'd first come in to try cryo, and that was really invigorating, but after a few sessions I wasn't sure that it was reducing the soreness and fatigue in my muscles. I tried the infrared sauna, though, and for whatever reason that was effective on me, so that's what I do."

There's no therapy at Restore—or anywhere else, for that matter—that will help anyone and everyone magically and immediately recover from every consequence of vigorous exercise. That hasn't stopped a lot of people from making outlandish claims about the myriad interventions that permit the body to return to a full state of energy and readiness after exercise, training, or competition, and it was those sorts of claims that got the attention of a journalist and lifelong endurance athlete named Christie Aschwanden.

As a high school track star, and later as a professional cyclist during her time as a college student, Aschwanden had never thought much about athletic recovery. But as she got a bit older—and as the science of recovery became big business around the world, in part due to many of those outlandish claims—it became one of the only things she thought about all the time. That's what prompted her to spend several years researching the subject for her 2019 book *Good to Go*.

"I'm a skeptic by nature," she wrote, "but as I've found myself needing more recovery time, those ads for recovery tools have begun to seem much more intriguing. I wanted to know: Do any of these products actually work?"[10]

The answer, Aschwanden found, was "yes" in some cases, "no" in plenty of others, and a resounding "it depends" in many more. Ultimately, she wrote, athletic recovery comes down to a simple principle: Listen to your own body.

Your body knows what it needs. It tells you when it provides immediate palpable feelings of betterment—more energy that can be invested in taking other steps on the virtual cycle. What we've done at Restore (and what we encourage everyone to do as they work toward hyper wellness in one of our studios, somewhere else, or in their own home) is to use the nine elements as a starting point for personal exploration. What makes you feel less fatigue and reduced soreness? What helps you heal from an injury faster? What leaves you feeling as though you have more energy than you had before, so you can return to an optimal level of activity sooner than you could have otherwise?

Your body knows what it needs.

Well, that's the right intervention for you.

What this means is that you might find there is something you can do for your own recovery that you cannot find at Restore. We're OK with that. We haven't cornered the market on everything that works for everyone, and we don't really intend to.

Deep tissue massage is one of many well-known examples of an intervention for athletic recovery that we're not doing at Restore. Researchers have repeatedly demonstrated that massage is an effective way to reduce the onset of muscle soreness,[11] decrease inflammation,[12] and improve a return to a full range of motion.[13] We didn't decide to not include massage therapy at Restore because it doesn't work; we didn't include it because it's already widely available in other places, and our goal has always been to fill the gaps in what most people can access.

To that end, there are six therapies that—pursuant to the weight of the scientific evidence—we have invested in that specifically target exercise recovery.

If you've read the chapter on cold therapy, you know that cryotherapy has been shown to promote reductions in muscle soreness, muscle damage, and inflammatory markers, as well as improvements in muscle strength. One meta-analysis, including nearly 40 randomized controlled trials with more than 1,200 participants, demonstrated that while cryo-based interventions don't work for every person in every situation, the vast majority of these studies showed statistically significant impacts.[14]

Likewise, as you know if you have already read the chapter on heat, sauna has been shown to improve circulation, reduce inflammation, and enhance immune function after a workout, and several studies of infrared sauna have demonstrated an intriguing reduction in creatine kinase, a key marker of muscle damage.[15] There's also some compelling evidence that infrared sauna can be effective at improving sleep—which is an element of hyper wellness on its own but also a key component of athletic recovery.[16]

Many of our clients additionally use IV drips specifically for exercise recovery, since this therapy can help replenish electrolytes and nutrients lost during exercise, reduce inflammation, and provide a quick energy boost. While the research that supports the effectiveness of intravenous hydration and nutritional supplementation for myriad health challenges is robust, the research specific to athletic recovery is still nascent. As recently as 2017, the National Athletic Trainers' Association argued that IV fluids are rarely necessary for hydration when water and sports drinks are readily available,[17] although it's worth noting that many of that association's members—including sports medicine and performance officials for professional sports teams across the United States—have publicly acknowledged their athletes' use of these therapies.

You might also recall that red, near-infrared, and infrared therapy have been demonstrated to be effective at limiting inflammation and promoting tissue repair,[18] findings that align with the experiences of many Restore clients.

Hyperbaric oxygen has also been demonstrated to have these impacts, likely through a decrease in inflammatory cell infiltration and a lowering of pro-inflammatory cytokines.[19]

Finally, compression therapy is one of the most popular for athletic recovery, and much of that interest has been driven by the long-term and successful use of this therapy by professional athletes and their trainers.

LeBron James played a big role in the compression revolution. Back in 2011, James was one of the most dominant forces in basketball, but his team, the Miami Heat, had been upset in the NBA Finals by the Dallas Mavericks, and James went back home to Akron, Ohio, to train for the next season. After one particularly hard workout, a trainer advised him to try out a computerized full-leg compression boot. "I'm always open to things that can help," James later explained. "I started using it, my legs started feeling better and I didn't stop. I started taking it on the road and everything. I mean, I think it's awesome."[20]

The year after James started using compression, his team was back in the Finals—this time with a resounding win.

It wasn't long before players from every team in the NBA were following his example, and soon computerized compression devices were in the training rooms of the world's best football, hockey, and soccer clubs, too.

Compression itself isn't anything new. Athletes have long used bandages and elastic sleeves following strenuous exercise, and many studies have demonstrated the overall beneficial impact on muscle soreness, fatigue, and strength,[21] which researchers generally attribute to the ways in which pressure influences blood circulation, which of course is vital for delivering oxygen to our muscles. But as computerized compression has gained popularity, many athletes have added it to their "athletic recovery rotation."

Lysa's personal circuit, for instance, includes compression, cryotherapy, red light therapy, and an IV drip that includes taurine, L-carnitine, B-complex, and glutamine.

"I started kickboxing just to stay in shape, never intending to ever fight anyone," she told us when we met her in Charlotte, North Carolina, about six months into a heavy cycle of training and roughly a month before her first amateur fight. "But the better I got, the more I wanted to test myself, so I started training harder and harder, and there was this moment when I wanted to know if I had the courage to step into the ring."

"The better I got, the more I wanted to test myself, so I started training harder and harder."

What Lysa learned during that period of training—and what we've heard from countless people who are training at their absolute peaks—is that the combinatory effects of multiple therapies appear to accentuate any singular benefits. "It's the thing where 'the whole is greater than its parts,'" Lysa said. "I did just compression every week for a month or so, and it was a big help, but I learned more about cryo and together it was better, so then I got really intrigued about what else would work, so now I come in once a week, and I'm doing two things each time I come in."

Built to Move

Our muscles make up about 40 percent of our body weight and contain up to three-quarters of all the proteins in our bodies. All that is for one important purpose: movement. And yet here we are in a world in which few people get the exercise they need, and our entire society has been set up in a way that discourages movement.

We must fight back! That can start for anyone—from couch potatoes to athletes in near-peak physical shape—by simply accentuating the physical movement already happening in their lives. The next step—which, again, is something that anyone can do regardless of their level of fitness—is to identify opportunities to convert inactivity to activity. We cannot forget, however, that no amount of motion is enough to keep pushing us toward hyper wellness without vigorous exercise. And with vigorous exercise comes a need for a personal regimen of recovery.

Any one of these principles can bring a person closer to their peak potential state of fitness. Combined, though, they represent one of the most powerful ways to arrive at that goal as soon as possible.

And if that's not a good enough reason to get moving, we don't know what is.

chapter 11

connection

You might have noticed the nod to Billy Joel's "Piano Man" in the introduction to this book when we spoke about "the regular crowd" who were lined up at one of the Restore studios in Austin. The cast of characters in Joel's song—John "at the bar," and Paul the "real estate novelist," and the waitress who was "practicing politics"—were all based on the regular crowd at the Executive Room, a bar on Wilshire Boulevard in Los Angeles where Joel had a regular gig as a piano player in the early 1970s. The singer has noted in interviews that he's not actually fond of the song, but he keeps singing it because he knows his fans love it—because it speaks to the innate human need to feel as though we belong.

We are hard-wired to connect with one another. It's a deeply embedded part of our evolutionary programming as a species that survived, and ultimately thrived, only because it was so very tribal. This continues to impact our lives today: People who feel well connected to friends, family members, and community suffer far lower rates of virtually every kind of chronic condition.[1]

We are hard-wired to connect with one another. It's a deeply embedded part of our evolutionary programming.

But here's the other thing that positive interpersonal connection does for us: It helps us feel better right away.

Grab a coffee with a friend. Hug your child. Garden with a neighbor. Go for a walk with your partner. If you were able to measure the biochemical composition of your body during any of those activities, what you would see is an immediate spike in oxytocin, a hormone that is associated with reduced stress and anxiety. You'd also likely see an increase in dopamine, a neurotransmitter known for its role in feelings of pleasure and motivation. And there would more than likely be a rise in serotonin, another neurotransmitter that contributes to happiness and a sense of well-being.[2] These are all feel-better responses that allow people to do more, so it was obvious to us that connection itself was an essential element of hyper wellness.

None of the elements of hyper wellness are exclusive to Restore, and this one least of all. Yet we still wanted our studios to be a place where people could mitigate the headwinds that prevent connection, and accentuate the tailwinds that promote it. So we knew we needed every studio to be a place in which people would feel as though they are part of a community, particularly because they are recognized as friends first and clients second.

That's the feeling that Tori says she gets when she walks into the Restore studio she visits each week in University Park, Florida. The professional track and field athlete told us that being a regular is akin to being part of the regular crowd at a local gym, coffee shop, or café. "Everybody knows my name when I come in," she said, "and that just feels amazing."

We've also worked hard to make sure that—within the reasonable bounds of space, privacy, and safety—the therapies we offer can be experienced alongside other people. The IV drip room is a good place to see this principle in action. It often feels more like a living room filled with friends than a place where people are "getting treatment." A lot of our clients always come in with a friend. Others have made "drip buddies," people they didn't know before spending an hour with them getting intravenous nutrients in side-by-side lounge chairs, and now schedule their appointments together.

During one recent afternoon at a studio in Omaha, Nebraska, we watched as two clients who had met for the first time bonded over their love for the Storm Chasers, a Minor League Baseball affiliate of the Kansas City Royals, and then hatched a plan together to take a road trip south to watch Vinnie Pasquantino, a first baseman who had been called up to the majors a season earlier.

When we checked in with Vic and Tyler a few weeks later, they confirmed that it wasn't just "IV talk."

"The Royals have been terrible this season," Tyler said, "but they happened to win that game, and Vinnie got a hit, so we had a great time and we're planning on doing it again later in the season."

Clearly, many clients are finding connection at Restore. But we'd be heartsick to learn our studios were the only place where that was happening in their lives, because connection can't just happen occasionally. It must be built into every part of our lives.

Connective Winds

The past few decades have seen many of our global societies fall into a tailspin of unconnectedness.

We've replaced real human relationships with something that social scientists call parasocial relationships—the psychological attachments that audience members have in mediated encounters with celebrities and online influencers. We've stopped talking to our friends and family members about politics—the shared problems of our lives—in favor of being told what to think by the endless parade of talking heads on 24-7 cable television programming and political podcasts. To make matters worse, a recent global pandemic left a lot of us scared to even be in the same room as another human being. And even when the most uncertain times of that pandemic were past us, a lot of people no longer even left their home to go to work as telecommuting became a norm in many industries.

Maybe you can say "That's not me," and if so then we're happy for you. But we're also willing to bet that you can't say "That's not anyone I know" or "That's not someone I deeply care about," which means that this world is a place where your connections with others have been strained, even if you have managed to avoid some of the worst traps and pitfalls of our modern culture.

It might seem like the easiest way to solve these problems would be to simply spend less time with virtual people and more time with actual people. But our proximity to living, breathing, human beings is only part of the problem because it doesn't do us any good to be around people if those people exert a toxic influence on our life.

So, the solution to addressing the headwind of disconnection isn't just reconnection, it's meaningful and positive connection. It's true friendship. It's having a partner you love, trust, and want to do amazing things with. It's having coworkers who share your values. It's having neighbors who have your back. And if that sounds like a lot of work, it's because it is. It takes a lot of energy to maintain healthy connections.

It doesn't do us any good to be around people
if those people exert a toxic influence on our life.

That's why we've come to believe the first step toward improving the connectivity we feel with others is to focus on ourselves. And yes, we understand how ridiculous that sounds, but think about it: If you don't have any energy to put *into* building healthy relationships, you'll never achieve a healthy relationship. Not with your friends. Not with your family members. Not with your coworkers or your neighbors. Before you can work on any of those things, you need energy—and the only way to get more energy is to invest in the virtuous cycle.

For instance, you might choose to build energy through healthy stressors like cold and heat therapies, thus priming your body for better rest, thus creating capacity to get more exercise. And it might not be until that point—several rotations of the virtuous cycle from where you began—that you have the energy it will take to do something that has the potential to build up a meaningful interpersonal connection, like making the effort to help a neighbor in need, deciding to begin physically going into the office a few days a week, asking someone out on a date, or reconnecting with a family member with whom you've fallen out of touch.

Most people generally have some, if not many, opportunities to deepen existing healthy connections. A coworker you already enjoy hanging out with. A parent you love visiting. A neighbor who enjoys cooking barbecue as much as you enjoy eating it. These are relational tailwinds and they take less energy to stoke, but there's still an investment to be made and, like any investment, a little smart nurturing goes a long way. To that end, it's good to recognize that connection, just like the other eight elements of hyper wellness, can be a powerful accentuator of wellness all by itself, but it's even more powerful when stacked up with other elements.

Just as there are tremendous benefits in using cold *and* heat therapies, bringing together breathing *and* hydration interventions, and utilizing rest *and* light *and* nourishment *and* movement, when we connect any of these elements to connection, we get an added boost.

Healthy stressors like cold and heat are powerful propellants of wellness, but experiencing these stresses with someone is a force multiplier. Indeed, we've noticed that people who show up for the first time to do cryotherapy with someone else are far more likely to come back again and again, even if they often come back alone. They began their journey with connection.

Rest is powerful and important. But there's a reason why humans choose partners and those partners almost always sleep together. Connection can make sleep better.

Movement is vital to our well-being. But time and again, studies have shown that the thing most effective at getting people to engage in vigorous exercise is being part of a community of people who are engaged in that activity together.[3]

There's no perfect prescription for better connection. As we've noted again and again, everyone is different. But there are some archetypes. There are those who have few if any real human connections and need to build more. There are those who have plenty of connections, but some if not many of those relationships are toxic. There are those who have a number of healthy relationships but could benefit from strengthening those connections. The truth is that most of us have some combination of these patterns in our life: We might have some connections but not enough, a number of toxic relationships we need to shed, and a few connections we would like to strengthen—if only we had the energy to do so.

So, let's take these "types" one at a time.

Building New Connections

Hunter was one of the most gifted networkers we'd ever met. A native of Austin, he'd started his first business in his teens and never stopped building, selling, having new ideas, and going through the process all over again. But one day in the early summer of 2022, over a beer at a tailgate party hosted by a mutual acquaintance, he confided that he didn't feel like he had any close friends.

Actually, "confided" might be the wrong word. It was a little bit like he was just saying it, matter-of-factly, as if he was simply relating a challenge one of his businesses was facing.

"I've actually tried to make friends over the years," he said. "I don't think I'm unlikable, but I'd understand if I'm not much fun for people to hang out with, if they think I'm boring or whatever because I'm usually pretty singularly focused on my work."

It's true that Hunter was focused in that way, but he was a good story-teller and a good listener, too. That's friendship material! What he didn't have—and what we suspected he may have never had before, given that he had fallen into entrepreneurship at an early age—was the extra energy it takes to nurture a new friendship. And since he was in his late 30s—a time in many people's lives when new families, rather than new friendships, are the priority—it was likely that he was going to have to invest a bit of energy into the process if he was indeed serious about building some meaningful relationships in his life.

Plunge-tub ice baths were growing popular in Austin at that time, and Hunter had recently put one in his home hoping to slow down the effects of aging that he was beginning to feel. "It's such a rush," he said. "I feel so awake and alive for hours afterward, and then I sleep so well that night, so the next day I feel more energy, too."

But what was he using all that energy for? To do even more work.

In our way of thinking, that was a missed opportunity. We'd never undercut the importance of work. It can be a place to find purpose, which is also beneficial to our long-term health and well-being.[4] But Hunter seemed to have purpose under control. What he appeared to be lacking was connection.

If you're similarly lacking connection—even if it's not to the extent that Hunter seemed to have been—it's likely going to be important for you to build up a reservoir of energy, and then make the difficult decision to invest that energy in the hard work of relationship building. A plunge in an ice tub can drive more work, sure, but it also could offer the energy it takes to decide to join a club, meet a neighbor, or begin dating.

Of course, cold therapy doesn't have to be the way you build that res-ervoir. Photobiomodulation has been shown to have great potential for increasing energy.[5] Good rest is obviously another way to increase capacity in this way. And exercise doesn't just take energy, it produces it!

But this is true of connection, too. Whether platonic[6] or romantic,[7] new, healthy relationships are often associated with feelings of increased energy—currency that can be spent on the virtuous cycle.

We're not going to hold forth on how to make friends. There have been plenty of books on that subject—and pretty much every children's television program has covered the basics: Be kind to others,[8] be your genuine self,[9] build upon mutual interests,[10] respect differences.[11] This isn't the book that's going to teach you how to be better at these things.

But you cannot do *any* of these things without building up your reservoir of energy. So that, truly, is the first step to building new connections.

Disconnecting from Toxicity

As hard as it can be to build connection when it's lacking, it's even more difficult to sever connections that are in place, even when we know those connections are taking more energy *from us* than they are giving *to us*.

Just about everyone has some experience with this: A friend, romantic partner, coworker, or other relationship that initially seemed to bring something valuable to your life turned out to come with a lot of baggage that shifted the equation. Suddenly, you were not gaining but giving energy—lots of it! You knew it was happening. And yet either you didn't act to create a healthy distance or you didn't do it soon enough.

There's no shame in this. It's also part of our evolutionary programming. For our ancient ancestors, social connections were so important to survival that the risk of severing a relationship was greater than the risk of staying in one. So it was that "breaking things off" was an experience that became painful.

"The things that cause us to feel pain are things that are evolutionary recognized as threats to our survival," social scientist Matthew Lieberman explained in 2013, the same year his seminal book on connection, *Social*, was first published, "and the existence of social pain is a sign that evolution has treated social connection like a necessity, not a luxury."[12]

It's not always easy to know when a relationship has begun to take more than it gives—a major sign of toxicity. After all, there's an energetic ebb and flow to *any* relationship. That's healthy. And the longer we've maintained a relationship—and the deeper the healthy ties once were—the lengthier these ebbs and flows may be. A lifelong friend who is going through a bad divorce and who needs your shoulder for support isn't necessarily a toxic friend.

There are a few important signs, though, that toxicity has entered the equation and that the energy exchange is increasingly unlikely to ever rebalance itself. One of these signs is respect; if someone you're connected to doesn't respect your needs, your time, and your stated boundaries, you're unlikely to ever be getting as much as you get from that relationship. Another is support; even if a person needs you more than you need them in the present moment, they should demonstrate that they care about the challenges you are facing just as much as you care about the challenges they are facing. Again, there are good books specific to this subject. (Antony Felix's *How To Stop Being Toxic*, while ostensibly a self-help guide for people who are toxic, is actually a savvy primer on how to identify "energy vampires.") A good rule of thumb in the context of the virtuous cycle, though, is a simple question: "Do I get an immediate, positive boost from my interactions with this person?" Even when someone needs you more than you need them, you should still be walking away from those experiences feeling better about yourself. "I helped a friend today and they appreciated it" is a powerful virtuous tailwind. "I tried to help and they made me feel like trash" is an even more powerful headwind.

*Even when someone needs you more than you
need them, you should still be walking away
from those experiences feeling better about yourself.*

Building healthy barriers between ourselves and toxic connections isn't easy. A toxic boss or coworker is a problem that almost always requires a change in one's job, which isn't something that can happen overnight and is notoriously stressful and exhausting.[13] Ending a toxic familial relationship or long-term friendship can mean abandoning decades of investment in a person who we've loved and will always love; there will certainly be a long and even lifelong period of mourning involved in this decision.[14]

The common denominator is energy: Without enough of it, severing ourselves from toxic connections can be impossible. So, to get to the point where we have enough energy to end these associations, we must build capacity through the virtuous cycle. And the good news is that each step we take toward hyper wellness helps us deal with the toxicity until such a time as we can take the big step of stepping away.

Strengthening Connections

Every part of your life should be supported by connections that contribute to your journey toward hyper wellness.

Work isn't supposed to be easy (if it was, we wouldn't call it "work" and we wouldn't need to pay people for it), but at the end of the day we should feel strengthened by the outcomes of our efforts. Friends and family members are going to need us sometimes more than we need them, but even when we are providing support to those we love, we are entitled to feel good about ourselves. The communities in which we live will never be free of drama (Robert Frost wrote that "good fences make good neighbors"), but it's not unreasonable to expect the people who live around you to share some basic notions of what it means to be neighborly.

Just as someone who is in excellent physical shape can always continue to take actions that move them even closer to a state of hyper wellness, there are always opportunities to strengthen our bonds with loving family, supportive friends, collaborative coworkers, and genial neighbors. In fact, this is one of the best places to generate capacity in times when you might feel as though you have plateaued on your journey toward hyper wellness.

For instance, because coworkers are often already proximal and present in our lives (many people spend more time with their workmates than they do with their immediate family members), the investment required to accentuate an already positive "work friendship" is minimal. It's an invitation to take a walk together on a lunch break. It's an unsolicited offer to help with a project. It's a suggestion to grab a drink or a meal after work.

Because we are already so invested in our family members and closest friends—and often understand them better than anyone else in our lives—it's relatively easy to strengthen already healthy connections. It's recognizing something happening in the community that a sibling might like to do and inviting them to do it with you. It's making an extra coffee date with your best friend. It's surprising your mother with another phone call.

And because in most cases we live closer in proximity to our neighbors than our friends or extended family members, it's not hard to identify opportunities to build upon these connections if those relationships are already friendly and supportive. It's arriving at a neighbor's door with some extra vegetables from your garden. It's lending a hand when you see someone painting their fence. It's simply checking in on matters beyond the courteous but vapid "How are you doing?"

Unlike building new connections or severing toxic ones, this takes little investment of energy. It requires you to identify a relational tailwind and then turn your sail in the slightest of directions to allow it to fill your sails.

Connecting the Elements

When we feel connected to the people around us, it accentuates the power of the other elements of hyper wellness. It helps us feel mindful about the world, gaining energy through experiencing what is happening around us rather than expending energy by judging or attempting to change things we cannot control. It helps us maintain a positive mood, allowing us to conserve energy for the things we want to do in life rather than expending it in a never-ending effort to restabilize our emotional state. It reduces stress, allowing our bodies to do what they are designed to do, rather than sending out a constant stream of biochemical alerts to be "on guard" against every possible social and physical affront.

As such, connection might best be thought of as the glue that binds our ability to engage in the other elements of hyper wellness.

That doesn't mean it's the most important element. Or even that it's the element that you should work on generating capacity from first. As we've noted, you might need to move through a few rotations of the virtuous cycle before you can hope to improve upon this part of your holistic wellness. But we beg you not to put off connection forever. In our way of seeing the world, there is no point in engaging with *any* of the other elements if the improvements that happen as a result do not lead to more meaningful, supportive, and joyful relationships.

Connection might best be thought of as the glue that binds our ability to engage in the other elements of hyper wellness.

We are, after all, designed to be connected, and so connection is both an element of hyper wellness and the entire point of it.

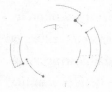

chapter 12

watchpoints and waypoints

Toward the beginning of this book, we asked you to take a journey throughout your entire body, feeling your way along every square inch of your being for pain and discomfort, tiredness and mental fogginess, stiffness and immobility—anything that might not be quite as it was at some point in your past.

We've noticed that when people evaluate their bodies in this deliberate way, they begin to recognize problems they had forgotten were problems and long accepted as "just part of life"—especially as they experience aging. What's more, they've given in to the idea that these issues are going to get worse over time. The pain will increase. The fatigue will, too. Mobility will diminish. Their overall sense of wellness will endlessly decline.

If we think of our future in that way, this census of our wellness can be something of a sad exercise, for it's a reckoning of many things that are wrong and will ostensibly get worse. But if we simply start by believing that there's *something* that can be done *somewhere* to address one of the many challenges that we identify, this exercise provides a concrete starting place from which to begin mitigating headwinds and accentuating tailwinds in the process that leads to hyper wellness. This permits us to embrace every moment, enjoying the small, right-away victories that happen along the way that are essential to this approach to wellness. From there, we can build from an ever-expanding base of contentedness, realizing long-term goals through these short-term gains.

When people do that, something amazing happens: This list of problems stops being a reminder of what's wrong and starts being a reckoning of what's possible. Improvements in one area beget capacity, capacity begets improvements in other areas, the list gets shorter, and even the issues that remain become less severe. The result is more energy. And yes, that energy can be spent targeting other problems—and some of it should be used in that way—but it can also be used for other things that improve our lives, those that bring us the greatest joy.

A walk with a cherished friend. A dinner with a loved one. A hike in the woods. A bike ride to a place you've never explored. A concert, a ball game, a dance, a picnic. A goal you've set aside or even given up on. An ambition you never would have even thought to have had in the first place. A life that's as long and as healthy and as happy as it can possibly be.

Of course, the specifics of what you do with the energy you gain during your hyper wellness journey are up to you. The only way you can screw it up is to not spend these newfound riches doing more of the things you love.

For the most part, the people we know who live life on the virtuous cycle are very able to identify how doing things that make them feel better right away contributes to improved long-term wellness. They remember how their knee felt a year ago and they know how it feels now. They recall the exhaustion they had back then and can describe the surplus of energy they have today. They have lived through a transformational change, and it's hard to miss the impact.

It's nonetheless still good, now and again, to go back to that original exercise. To move deliberately from your toes to your head, taking stock of what you find.

When a friend of ours did this, he was amazed by what he discovered. "There are things I've intentionally worked on over the past year that I knew had improved," Kris said. "My back problems were the center of my attention during that time, and just lying there, working my way up my spine, the difference was so clear—but that's what I expected. What I didn't realize was how much these other parts of my body, these little aches and pains that I had been carrying around for so long, had been reduced as well."

By way of example, Kris rolled his shoulders forward and back, like a baseball pitcher loosening up before a game. "Last year when I would do this, there was this gravelly sensation and a small amount of pain, but it was almost imperceptible compared to the pain I was always feeling in my back, so I didn't even appreciate it as a problem," he said. "Now my shoulders move freely. No roughness in motion. No pain at all. I didn't set out to work on this. It just happened. And I wouldn't have even realized it if I hadn't taken stock of everything last year and then done it again now."

If you engage in this exercise, you're also likely to identify improvements in wellness that you didn't intentionally set out to fix, just as Kris did. Alas, any honest assessment will also result in the discovery of some challenges that weren't there before; most of us can't get through any lengthy period of life without a few new bumps and bruises after all! That just allows for a new road map. A few new targets. A few new goals. A few more opportunities to put the nine elements of hyper wellness to work in different ways. To make you physically stronger. To make you emotionally more resilient. To make you mentally sharper. And to drive you toward a life of less negative stress, a greater sense of balance, a renewed thirst for discovery, and a journey that takes you to your greatest potential.

A few new targets. A few new goals. A few more opportunities to put the nine elements of hyper wellness to work in different ways.

And yes, as we've admitted before, we'd love it if you found your way to this future by way of one of our studios. But we want to reiterate that you don't have to. We've made it easy to access a lot of the therapeutic tools that research has demonstrated are likely to result in immediate improvements to people's health. But we haven't cornered the market on this stuff, and we don't want to. Competition is healthy, and when people identify their own ways of engaging these elements, they reveal opportunities for even more people to pursue the goal of hyper wellness.

But whether you go on this journey at a Restore studio, somewhere else, or on your own, there are certain things you need to know to make sure you're moving safely, smartly, and steadily in the right direction.

Assessing Safety and Success

Tori, the track and field athlete we first mentioned in chapter 11, once told us that when she leaves a cryotherapy session, "It feels like I can bounce again."

We're so lucky that Tori has chosen to be part of our community, but the truth is that a big part of that relationship is nothing more than geography: There just happened to be a Restore studio near where Tori trains. As much as we are driven to open centers across the United States and around the world, it's going to take some time to reach that goal. So, for now, there are a lot of people whose only choice for cryo is to go somewhere *other* than a Restore studio.

If that's your situation, it's important to know what you're getting. Done under the wrong circumstances, after all, cryotherapy can be dangerous. Each year, we hear stories of people who suffered burns as a result of coming into direct contact with liquid nitrogen or its vapors, a result of poorly designed or malfunctioning chambers.

Different countries and US states regulate cryotherapy in various ways, and this patchwork of laws means you shouldn't assume there's a uniform level of safety being met by every cryo provider. The same is true to a greater or lesser extent when it comes to every other therapy we've mentioned in this book. There are risks to ice baths, light therapy at every wavelength and level of intensity, IV hydration, nutritional supplementation, and hyperbaric oxygen.

So, your safety is in your hands. As such, here's what you should be looking for:

Complete transparency: No matter what kind of therapy you are seeking, the place you go should allow you to tour the facility before signing up for treatment, and any questions you have about safety should be knowledgeably answered. Staff members shouldn't seem put out by your questions. And if they don't have an immediate answer, they should seem eager to identify someone within their organization who does. Follow-up questions shouldn't be treated as burdensome—especially when those questions are about safety.

No-pressure sales: You shouldn't be pressured to do anything you're not comfortable doing. It's fine and even good for staff members to suggest services that might additionally help you reach your goals, but you shouldn't be made to feel as though you're making a mistake or wasting someone's time by declining such an opportunity. Therapies that work will sell themselves through a growing assemblage of peer-reviewed research and the experiences of people who have gone before you. Pressure tactics are for snake-oil salesmen.

Cleanliness: Some health centers feel like fancy spas. Others feel like a doctor's office. Still others look like tanning salons. No matter the aesthetic, though, the maintenance of hygienic conditions is a must. Business owners who are inattentive to cleanliness are almost always cutting corners in other ways, too.

Realistic expectations: There's no panacea for every illness, and there's no therapy in the world that will change your life in one session. While we believe that therapies aligned to the nine elements can absolutely make many people feel better in some meaningful way—either during or soon after their first treatment—we would never suggest any of these things have the power to change a person's life in one session. So, an introductory session of any type of therapy should make you feel better in some meaningful way, but that's a *step* onto the virtuous cycle that leads to long-term wellness, not a one-and-done elixir. Anyone claiming anything beyond that doesn't care for your short- or long-term wellness.

Safety: Only about half of the cryo chambers in commercial use right now are "closed systems," in which there's no way for nitrogen to come in contact with a user's body. Nitrogen itself isn't bad, per se—indeed, although we've been instrumental in a push for electric chambers, we still use nitrogen-cooled machines in many of our centers—but we would never personally step into an open system, in which *any* amount of nitrogen is released inside or around the chamber. Even in a closed system, though, you must be able to leave the chamber at any time without someone's assistance. You should also be able to contact a staff member when you are receiving treatment—and this is true for every therapy that aligns to one of the nine elements of hyper wellness. If you cannot access help when you need it, you are in a dangerous situation.

Privacy: Most people do cryotherapy, red light therapy, and sauna in naked or nearly naked conditions. No matter what size or shape you are, your body is beautiful—but it's yours and yours alone to share or not share with others. You should never have to argue for a level of privacy that makes you comfortable; it should be a given. You should also feel empowered to ask questions and get straight answers about how any personal health information you provide in order to access a therapy will be protected.

Reviews: Many of the therapies people use in alignment with the nine elements of hyper wellness can be uncomfortable in some way. You'll not be shocked to learn, for instance, that cryotherapy is very cold and saunas are very warm—and not everyone likes being really cold or really hot. People who have claustrophobia might not be comfortable with hyperbaric oxygen treatment. And even when a therapy itself doesn't bother someone, there are times in which misunderstandings or mistakes result in a customer feeling as though they didn't get what they paid for. These sorts of things can happen in the best of situations, and we live in a world in which anyone can write a negative public review for anything for any reason. Broadly speaking, though, the weight of all reviews should reflect positive customer experiences in which people feel they were treated with respect, received a service that was commensurate with what they paid, and are excited to come again.

Your safety is in your hands.

What to Watch For

By the time you read this book, many innovations that were little more than wistful ideas when we were writing it will have emerged as potent strategies for improving healthspans and lifespans. Studies that were underway will have given us a clearer picture of how to use these practices to help people in a variety of circumstances. Many of the newer therapies we were investigating could be being offered in a Restore studio near you. That's how fast things are moving.

Peptides are a great example of how quickly the technology and research landscape can change. At the time we began writing this book, these short chains of amino acids were just barely popping onto our own personal radars. But we are constantly evaluating emerging products and services and, by the time this book is in your hands, we suspect that there will be even more interest and enthusiasm around these molecules, which can help regulate hormone levels, impact cellular signaling, and modulate immune responses.

The first-ever synthetic peptide is one that you have absolutely heard of, and one that has likely touched the life of someone you love: insulin, which was first shown to be effective at reducing blood glucose way back in 1922. But even though this drug has improved the lives of hundreds of millions of people in the century that has passed since then, a surprisingly small number of other peptides were approved for the rest of the 20th century, mainly because it turns out that insulin, which is relatively easy to produce, is an outlier. Other peptides proved very hard to make. But peptide development has entered a new era in the past few years as advances in structural biology, new techniques for synthesis, and new technologies for analysis have accelerated the development of these therapeutics. In the first few years of the 2020s, the US Food and Drug Administration has been on a tear, approving many new peptides for general use and even more for experimental use, with many users reporting quickly noticeable improvements in strength, exercise recovery, energy, libido, and focus.

Many Restore clients are already using one class of peptides, semaglutides, which mimic the natural processes that make us feel full after eating, regulate appetite and cravings, and improve blood sugar control. Restore's chief medical officer, Rich Joseph, a specialist in obesity and metabolic health, has used semaglutides for years in his practice and seen the positive effects these therapies can have on his patients' wellness. Now, emerging research is showing similarly impressive effects with other peptides to simulate and stimulate normal physiological processes, helping to improve metabolism, boost immune function, enhance cellular communication, aid in tissue repair and growth, reduce inflammation, protect against oxidative stress, and improve neural function. Meanwhile, peptides employed against specific diseases are showing promise for the treatment of diabetes, cardiovascular diseases, gastrointestinal diseases, cancer, and infectious diseases.[1]

Both of us have personally benefitted from peptide injections and, like many others in the health space, we have been spending a lot of time and energy on the challenge of bringing these therapies to people who need them. But this process takes time—and it should, especially when we're talking about something that science has suggested would be most effective if administered *inside* our client's bodies. It's frustrating to move slowly toward the goal of helping people, but safety is paramount. We have built up this business, after all, by asking our clients to trust us with the most important thing in their life, their wellness. We simply can't get things like this wrong.

All of this is to say that you shouldn't dismiss a potential treatment just because it wasn't in this book. But nor should you accept every new claim that comes along; there are plenty of people who are far more interested in lining their pockets in the short term than helping anyone, even themselves, live healthier and more joyful lives in the long term. With that in mind, here are the sorts of questions we'll be asking ourselves as we evaluate the potential of everything coming down the pike:

A hyper wellness fit: When you evaluate a potential health intervention through the lens of the feel-better-do-more cycle, it should simply make sense. The benefits should be palpable in the form of less pain, more mobility, or more energy, and the resulting capacity should be transferable to other actions that make your life better. It should also fit into the work you're already doing to move toward hyper wellness. We encourage exploration of alternatives that may be easier to do, more effective for you as an individual, or less expensive, but any change should be easily integrated into the regimen that has kept you on the virtuous cycle up to that point.

Safety and success: If you search through this book, you won't find the word *proven* in relation to any of the studies we've cited in support of the therapies we believe can have the greatest impact on people's lives. Everything we do is guided by science, but science doesn't give us proof; it gives us evidence, and we can use that evidence to make decisions guided by informed expectations. What we've tried to do in our own lives, and what we'll continue to do as we explore new opportunities to accentuate the virtuous cycle, is to identify interventions that have the greatest reward-to-risk ratio. Sauna is a great example: Humans have thousands of years of experience with this therapy and nearly a century of modern scientific research. And what has been shown is that it's an effective intervention that, when used in moderation, is very safe. By way of contrast, and as a rule, the newer an intervention is, the less we know about both safety and success. As such, we should be more cautious about keeping the "risk" side of that ratio very low—even if it appears that the "reward" side seems very high. Everyone will come to their own personal decisions about what balance is right for them—some people are more risk tolerant and others are more risk averse. If you're not sure, lean hard into safety.

Follow good shepherds: Many of the purported experts who have emerged in recent years and exerted tremendous influence over the health decisions of millions of followers don't look like they're faring so well themselves. That's a strange phenomenon. The people who guide the decisions we make about our own health should be living, breathing, walking, talking exhibits of the effectiveness of the interventions they recommend to others. To this end, active professional athletes can be good people to pay attention to, since they have a huge stake in being hyper well, but it's also important to recognize that many athletes will trade the future for the present (this is how we got Major League Baseball's "steroids era" in the 1990s and early 2000s). With that in mind, the individuals we're most likely to seek as guides in our lives are those who have a long history of "looking the part." But, of course, you shouldn't assume that just because someone looks young, fit, and healthy in a video or photo that they would appear that way if you saw them walking down the street. AI-enabled digital "de-aging" has long been used in Hollywood to make actors look decades younger, and is increasingly accessible for anyone who can afford a cheap piece of software. Photo filters and editing are even older and easier ways to make someone look younger and fitter than they are. And there are plenty of surgical interventions that can make it seem as though the ravages of aging didn't touch a person. So, how does one choose a "good shepherd"? Well, first remember that no one becomes "a specimen" by doing just one thing, and anyone who says otherwise is getting paid to say so. Second, understand that while there's nothing wrong with someone getting paid to endorse a product, if a person wasn't using that product until they were being paid, then the payment was more influential to them than the product. Third, take some time to evaluate the example that someone you wish to emulate has set over time: Those who have been consistent in what they say and do for many years are far better stewards of your health than those whose long-term actions are difficult or impossible to pin down.

Fad in, fade out: Not a year goes by in which a fad health intervention doesn't pop quickly onto our radar screens—and then just as quickly blips out into the ether. And yet these fads often compel millions of people to waste their money, time, and energy on something that never had a shred of supporting evidence of success *or* safety. This happens again and again because people facing the reality of aging often feel they don't have a moment to waste. But if you're following a hyper wellness lifestyle—and particularly if you're not yet suffering from a vast accumulation of aging-related symptoms—you're *already* doing a lot to ensure a much longer and much healthier life. In essence, you've bought yourself time, and one of the greatest rewards for this hard work is the fact that you can afford to wait for fads to fade—or, of course, for therapies that actually work to be increasingly supported by research and experience.

You shouldn't dismiss a potential treatment just because it wasn't in this book. But nor should you accept every new claim that comes along, either.

Making Waypoints

One of the challenges of explaining how right-away interventions can promote long-term wellness is that there are plenty of things in our lives that can make us feel better in the short term but aren't at all helpful for accentuating wellness years down the road.

If you're feeling a little blue right now and someone you loved gave you a scoop of ice cream with hot fudge, whipped cream, and one of those neon-colored cherries, there's a pretty good chance that you'd feel a little bit better right away. But does ice cream build capacity as part of the virtuous cycle? Alas, it does not. Yet it's an enticing thought because—let's be honest—pretty much everyone likes a good ice cream sundae!

How do we separate things that accentuate both immediate and long-term wellness from those that only make us feel better in the present moment? The answers can be found in all the days, weeks, and months in between.

"When I started out, I was doing an IV drip every week, and then I tried to space it out a little more as I was able to do other things to feel better in addition to that," Christopher, the banking executive who we introduced in Chapter 9, told us. "Right now what I've learned is that two weeks is too long for me, and 10 days is just about right. So that's where I'm at, and that's helping sustain continued improvements in every part of my life."

While Christopher does walk away from each drip session feeling substantially better than he did when he walked in, he is also recognizing benefits sustained over the following week or so. What's more, the positive momentum—an overall sense of *consistently* improving wellness—is also being sustained from week to week and month to month. Also, as you might recall, those improvements have been reflected in the hard data he is getting from his semiannual blood tests.

These are the sorts of intermediate assessments—waypoints of wellness, so to speak—that can help guide our decision-making on a long voyage. And this is important, because without such waypoints any journey is likely to become mired in disorientation.

Many people set chronological waypoints in their lives. Graduate high school by 18. Have a bachelor's degree by 22. Be making a certain amount of money by 30. Retire by 65. Onward it goes. And what happens when we miss these waypoints? Discouragement and disillusion!

Folks also tend to do this in their health journeys. Lose five pounds by next month. Be running a 10-minute mile by the New Year. Get down to a certain blood pressure level before the next doctor's appointment. And if we miss those waypoints, all too often we convince ourselves that we are incapable or even unworthy of wellness.

This is absolute madness! Do you know what happens when a young person who has hit a few rough patches in their life fails to graduate high school before they turn 19, but nonetheless keeps working toward that goal? That person eventually graduates from high school! And do you know what happens when someone keeps losing weight toward a long-term goal, but at a slower pace than they had hoped for? They eventually reach that goal.

The virtuous cycle works the same way. Sometimes it helps us reach a goal faster than we imagined we might, and that's wonderful. But other times it takes a little longer, and that's OK, because time matters far less than direction. If your pain is abating, your mobility is improving, your

fatigue is subsiding, or your energy is increasing, then the time it takes is
of far less consequence than the momentum you're building along the way,
even if that momentum is incremental.

---

*If your pain is abating, your mobility is improving, your
fatigue is subsiding, or your energy is increasing, then the
time it takes is of far less consequence than the momentum
you're building along the way.*

It's equally important to remember that your body is a system of systems, a place where improvements in any one area will pay dividends in
another. This is one of the reasons that one of the most common ways
to assess health—body weight—can be such a poor indicator of actual
wellness.

Macey, for example, began using cryotherapy in her late 40s, after
hearing from a friend that it could be helpful for mitigating menopausal
weight gain—a beneficial outcome that many of our clients have shared
and that is supported by emerging research, especially among women who
are also at increased risk of heart disease, stroke, and diabetes.[2]

"I think I'm like a lot of people in that the experience of getting that
cold is such a rush in and of itself, so I was hooked pretty quickly," she
said. "But I did it for several months and my weight didn't actually drop,
so that was sort of disappointing."

If weight was Macey's only waypoint, she might have given up. But she
also recognized an improvement in sleep in the nights following her cryo
sessions and a reduction in joint pain. "So, it occurred to me that even
though I had gone into this for weight loss, I was better off in other ways
for doing it, and that kept me going," she said.

Eventually, Macey did lose some weight. But that came after many
turns of the virtuous cycle—and seemingly not as a direct consequence of
the cryo, but rather as a result of the fact that she was able to reinvest her

reduced pain and improved restfulness into more exercise. Importantly, she didn't give up when she didn't see what she first expected to see. She kept her eyes open for other signs of success.

With just about every passing day, there are new ways to measure those other, unexpected successes—especially biomonitoring devices that can help you better understand how your decisions, activities, and therapies are affecting your wellness. There are rings and watches and patches and implants, and an increasing number of artificially intelligent programs that can alert you to what all the data those products are collecting is telling you in aggregate. Meanwhile, the cost for blood tests is falling, while the amount of meaningful and actionable information in those tests is going up. Don't be content with one waypoint!

Another way to think about this is to imagine yourself as ancient seafarer. You've been taught to navigate by the stars—to seek out a certain constellation and use it to set your heading. But it's cloudy on your current journey, and you are beginning to wonder whether you're headed in the right direction. Would you not utilize the light of the moon when it set the clouds aglow? Would you not use the sun as it rose, traveled across the sky, and set? And when the first signs of land appeared on the distant horizon, would you ignore that and keep looking to the night skies, waiting for the weather to change, so that you could make sure you were headed in the right direction using the signs you'd been *intending* to use? Of course not. We should not ignore waypoints telling us that we are getting better just because some are telling us nothing has changed.

Don't lose sight of the horizon by fretting over the stars.

Hyper wellness is a complex equation, but its most robust variables are simple and directional. Wellness is accentuated when pain is mitigated, mobility is improved, fatigue is reduced, and energy is increased. Other things can be influential to the equation, but a lack of change in any subvariable doesn't mean a loss of momentum toward the ultimate goal. If you're not losing ground in any other area, any gain puts you closer to balance, to fullness of energy, and to meeting the potential of what your body is capable of. Don't lose sight of the horizon by fretting over the stars.

Finding Your Why

Even if you can feel the benefits in the short term, see them in the medium term, and appreciate them in the long term, you will still likely find that the journey toward hyper wellness is long and, at times, difficult. It takes time and effort. It's not always comfortable and fun. And because we live in a world of abundance, indolence, and distraction, it's easy to slip up, lose momentum, and fall back on bad habits. And let us be frank here: If you don't believe these times will happen to you, you are at greater risk when they do.

So, please, accept this truth with open eyes and an open heart: At some point your hyper wellness journey will get hard, and you will need to dig deeper to maintain or regain your spot on the virtuous cycle. What some people think this means is that they will have to tap into a well of willpower, an internal source of energy that will keep them moving when times get tough and failure seems imminent. That's true in part, but there's one important caveat: That internal source of energy is almost never actually internal. It's almost always supplied by something external.

A child. A spouse. A friend. A goal that, if reached, will help others. A purpose!

These are the external things that drive internal fortitude, and that give us the energy we need to keep going when seemingly every other signal in life tells us to stop. And we should not wait until things are hard to go looking for these things. We should know from the start of our journey the answer to a simple question: Why?

This way, amid a struggle—when we ask, "Why am I doing this?"—it will take no energy at all to come up with the answer. It will be there, for it always has been there. It's something we can anchor onto.

Better than one "why" is two. Better than two is three. Having a re-dundancy of anchors is important, because our lives are long and change happens in unpredictable ways. And while we don't intend to be morbid, here, we do need to be honest: What anchors you today might not be there tomorrow, and if suddenly it's not, that might be the very reason that you are suddenly adrift in this journey, struggling to keep going, faltering with each attempted step, and falling behind.

So it is that "I am doing this so that I can be here for my partner" is a good start, but "I am doing this so I can be here for my partner and my children" is even better. These are, as it happens, the "whys" we hear most often from our clients, but there are endless others.

Chhay, a client from the central California valley, suffered through the end of his marriage and the death of his father in a single year. "It was a lot of change all at once, and I was feeling pretty aimless, and not interested in doing anything for my health."

Thankfully, Chhay still had a "why," a Buddhist church his family had been going to since he was very young. Recently, the church building was starting to show its age. It needed a lot of work. "It could take us years or maybe a decade to raise the money and do the work," Chhay said. "And I'm aware that it's going to take a lot of energy to do this while working and, hopefully at some point, finding a new partner and starting a family of my own. But at this dark moment in my life I've been able to lock onto that. I told myself, 'I need to have the energy to make this happen,' and that kept me working toward my health goals."

What makes it worthwhile for you to be healthier and want to *stay* healthier for a long time to come? It's important to ask this question and answer it—and to do so often. Don't wait for times to be difficult. Know the answers today. Remind yourself of those answers every day. And as life changes, accept that the answers will change, too. This will sustain you when you need it. And yes, you will need it.

The good news is that times won't always be tough. Even if you always have your "why" close at hand, you're not always going to need it. Indeed, the whole idea of the virtuous cycle is that, in most times, it's easy to keep going. One act creates capacity, permitting another act, and another, and away we go, collecting right-away benefits that coalesce into long-term wellness.

By all means, enjoy that momentum. Savor it. Even save some of it up. You deserve it.

Conclusion

We often think back to the days after we first experienced cryo-therapy—a period in which an idea began to form for taking something good and making it better.

That wasn't revolutionary. It was simply doing what we've always done. It's how we've built many successful companies during our professional lives.

But something changed shortly after we opened our first studio, as we met clients who turned into friends, and who shared with us their stories. They were feeling better. They were doing more. The life-transforming power of the virtuous cycle was revealing itself. We began to wonder why it was that this therapy—and the others we quickly began introducing at a growing number of studios across the country—hadn't been available to these people all along.

It has been clear to just about everyone, and for a long time, that the "sick care" model of health care delivery is irreparably broken. And yet the past few decades have brought few changes to a system that treats people as unworthy of care until they are sick or injured, and then often tells them there's not much that can be done to make things better.

Under this terrible status quo, the notion that accentuating holistic individual health can empower people to live closer to their absolute potential—to be hyper well—is treated as a radical and dangerous idea. "The system is just not ready for that concept," we've been told again and again.

Perhaps that's true. There are many reasons why "Big Medicine" is set up this way, some more flabbergasting than others, but the bottom line is that the dominant paradigm is firmly entrenched. So, we must accept that hyper wellness is a category of care almost completely in the hands of those who wish to live longer, healthier, and happier lives.

The fight is ours as individuals.

That doesn't mean we have to go into that fight blind. It's true that health research tends to focus on what can be done to help *sick* people recover more—or at least suffer less—but embedded in a vast library of peer-reviewed scientific journal articles are plenty of findings that can be applied to anyone's life to mitigate the headwinds and accentuate the tailwinds of wellness. We've cited hundreds of these studies in this book, and in doing so we've merely scratched the surface of an already compelling and fast-growing body of research that supports the transformative power of the nine elements of hyper wellness.

The research tells us that cold is a potent instigator of healthy stress. Heat is too. Oxygen is fundamental not simply to sustaining our lives but to ensuring every system in our body is thriving. Hydration is a devastatingly underappreciated mediator of wellness. Rest is a tremendous force multiplier. Light supports health and healing in numerous ways that we've only just begun to explore. Nourishment is patently vital to our well-being and yet all too often ignored or misunderstood. We are built to move, but we don't do it with enough purpose, vigor, and attentiveness to recovery. And as we connect these principles together, we are better able to connect with others, as well.

A journey to hyper wellness can start with any one of these elements, each of which has the potential to provide right-away benefits that expand our capacity to do more. There's no correct order of application, no perfect way to stack these principles upon one another. Eventually, though, we believe that *all* these elements should be a part of everyone's lives.

What happens when that happens? Well, the obvious outcome is an ever-improving state of physical wellness. Less pain, chronic disease, and aging. More mobility, energy, and resilience.

Upon that physical foundation, we can build greater emotional wellness. Less frustration and resentment. More contentedness and rationality.

When we have physical and emotional wellness, we are in a better position to improve upon our mental wellness. Less brain fog and burnout. More flexibility in thought, adaptability to change, and precision in ideas.

The final outcome is spiritual wellness—a growing ability to balance doing with being. Less fear, confusion, and self-doubt. More mindfulness, discipline, and discovery.

Picture yourself in your greatest possible state of physical, emotional, mental, and spiritual wellness. Whatever that looks like is what you are working toward. That's your horizon.

Picture yourself in your greatest possible state of physical, emotional, mental, and spiritual wellness.

Of course, upon every horizon is another. We've told you that hyper wellness is a goal that can be approached but never fully realized—that there's always more potential to identify and pursue. This is true. But this does not mean those who are on a hyper wellness journey are doomed to discontentedness. All evidence to the contrary; the many people we've come to know on this journey have shown us, again and again, the joy and satisfaction that comes from greater physical, emotional, mental, and spiritual wellness.

Do they also know there is more out there for them to accomplish? Yes. Every one of them. Professional athletes at the top of their games. Innovators from the world's top companies. Thought leaders in their fields.

Trailblazers on the front edges of progress. Spiritual guides who many others look to for enlightenment. We've yet to meet anyone who is on the path to hyper wellness who would say they have no further ways to feel better and no additional ways to do more of what they love. But this, as the saying goes, is "a feature, not a bug." For if there's one thing that seems to separate humans from the many millions of other animal species on this planet, it's that we are never content with what is.

We are always reaching.

We would like you to keep reaching. Whether you haven't yet introduced any of the nine elements into your life, are just beginning to, or have been doing so successfully for a long time, there's something more to reach for—and you are worthy of it.

No matter who you are.

No matter where you are.

No matter what obstacles you're facing.

You are worthy of being hyper well.

And the next step in that journey can be taken right here, right now, right away.

Notes

Introduction

1. Breasted, J. H. (1930). *The Edwin Smith Surgical Papyrus.*
2. Allan, R., Malone, J., Alexander, J., Vorajee, S., Ihsan, M., Gregson, W., Kwiecien, S., & Mawhinney, C. (2022). Cold for centuries: a brief history of cryotherapies to improve health, injury and post-exercise recovery. *European Journal of Applied Physiology.*

Chapter 1

1. Johnson, W. (Oct. 24, 1977). This strange and perilous joint. *Sports Illustrated.*
2. Ingram, J. G., Fields, S. K., Yard, E. E., & Comstock, R. D. (2008). Epidemiology of knee injuries among boys and girls in US high school athletics. *American Journal of Sports Medicine.*
3. Whitaker, K. L., Scott, S. E., Winstanley, K., Macleod, U., & Wardle, J. (2014). Attributions of cancer "alarm" symptoms in a community sample. *PloS One.*
4. Jones R. C. (2004). History of the Department of Surgery at Baylor University Medical Center. *Proceedings (Baylor University. Medical Center).*
5. Blondin, A. (March 3, 2022). Ken Rideout wins Myrtle Beach Marathon to celebrate birthday. *The Sun News.*
6. Ruby, J. G., Wright, K. M., Rand, K. A., Kermany, A., Noto, K., Curtis, D., Varner, N., Garrigan, D., Slinkov, D., Dorfman, I., Granka, J. M., Byrnes, J., Myres, N., & Ball, C. (2018). Estimates of the heritability of human longevity are substantially inflated due to assortative mating. *Genetics.*

7. Barzilai, N. (Sept. 28, 2011). Healthy until 120. *Haaretz.*
8. Verducci F. M. (2000). Interval cryotherapy decreases fatigue during repeated weight lifting. *Journal of Athletic Training.*
9. Salas-Fraire, O., Rivera-Pérez, J. A., Guevara-Neri, N. P., Urrutia-García, K., Martínez-Gutiérrez, O. A., Salas-Longoria, K., & Morales-Avalos, R. (2023). Efficacy of whole-body cryotherapy in the treatment of chronic low back pain: quasi-experimental study. *Journal of Orthopaedic Science.*
10. Kelly, J., & Bird, E. (2021). Improved mood following a single immersion in cold water. *Lifestyle Medicine.*
11. Yildirim, N., Filiz Ulusoy, M., & Bodur, H. (2010). The effect of heat application on pain, stiffness, physical function and quality of life in patients with knee osteoarthritis. *Journal of Clinical Nursing.*
12. Selfe, T. K., & Taylor, A. G. (2008). Acupuncture and osteoarthritis of the knee: a review of randomized, controlled trials. *Family & Community Health.*
13. Selfe, T. K., & Innes, K. E. (2013). Effects of meditation on symptoms of knee osteoarthritis. *Alternative & Complementary Therapies.*
14. Ali, A., Rosenberger, L., Weiss, T. R., Milak, C., & Perlman, A. I. (2017). Massage therapy and quality of life in osteoarthritis of the knee: a qualitative study. *Pain Medicine.*
15. Liu, X., Machado, G. C., Eyles, J. P., Ravi, V., & Hunter, D. J. (2018). Dietary supplements for treating osteoarthritis: a systematic review and meta-analysis. *British Journal of Sports Medicine.*
16. Smeenk, H. E., Koster, M. J., Faaij, R. A., de Geer, D. B., & Hamaker, M. E. (2014). Compression therapy in patients with orthostatic hypotension: a systematic review. *Netherlands Journal of Medicine.*
17. Sellami, M., Bragazzi, N., Prince, M. S., Denham, J., & Elrayess, M. (2021). Regular, intense exercise training as a healthy aging lifestyle strategy: preventing DNA damage, telomere shortening and adverse DNA methylation changes over a lifetime. *Frontiers in Genetics.*
18. Susko, A. M., & Fitzgerald, G. K. (2013). The pain-relieving qualities of exercise in knee osteoarthritis. *Open Access Rheumatology: Research and Reviews.*

Chapter 2

1. Reber, K. C., König, H. H., & Hajek, A. (2018). Obesity and sickness absence: results from a longitudinal nationally representative sample from Germany. *BMJ Open.*
2. Chistiakov, D. A., Sobenin, I. A., Revin, V. V., Orekhov, A. N., & Bobryshev,

Y. V. (2014). Mitochondrial aging and age-related dysfunction of mitochondria. *BioMed Research International.*

3. Petersen, K. F., Befroy, D., Dufour, S., Dziura, J., Ariyan, C., Rothman, D. L., DiPietro, L., Cline, G. W., & Shulman, G. I. (2003). Mitochondrial dysfunction in the elderly: possible role in insulin resistance. *Science.*

4. Melton, L. J., 3rd, Khosla, S., Crowson, C. S., O'Connor, M. K., O'Fallon, W. M., & Riggs, B. L. (2000). Epidemiology of sarcopenia. *Journal of the American Geriatrics Society.*

5. Volpi, E., Nazemi, R., & Fujita, S. (2004). Muscle tissue changes with aging. *Current Opinion in Clinical Nutrition and Metabolic Care.*

6. Sun, N., Youle, R. J., & Finkel, T. (2016). The mitochondrial basis of aging. *Molecular Cell.*

7. Li, J., Bonkowski, M. S., Moniot, S., Zhang, D., Hubbard, B. P., Ling, A. J., Rajman, L. A., Qin, B., Lou, Z., Gorbunova, V., Aravind, L., Steegborn, C., & Sinclair, D. A. (2017). A conserved NAD+ binding pocket that regulates protein-protein interactions during aging. *Science.*

8. Berbudi, A., Rahmadika, N., Tjahjadi, A. I., & Ruslami, R. (2020). Type 2 diabetes and its impact on the immune system. *Current Diabetes Reviews.*

9. Glare, P. A., Davies, P. S., Finlay, E., Gulati, A., Lemanne, D., Moryl, N., Oeffinger, K. C., Paice, J. A., Stubblefield, M. D., & Syrjala, K. L. (2014). Pain in cancer survivors. *Journal of Clinical Oncology.*

10. Jack, K., McLean, S. M., Moffett, J. K., & Gardiner, E. (2010). Barriers to treatment adherence in physiotherapy outpatient clinics: a systematic review. *Manual Therapy.*

11. Marchese, D. (May 21, 2023) Want to live longer and healthier? Peter Attia has a plan. *New York Times.*

12. Blum, K., Han, D., Baron, D., Kazmi, S., Elman, I., Gomez, L. L., Gondre-Lewis, M. C., Thanos, P. K., Braverman, E. R., & Badgaiyan, R. D. (2022). Nicotinamide adenine dinucleotide (NAD+) and enkephalinase inhibition (IV1114589NAD) infusions significantly attenuate psychiatric burden sequalae in substance use disorder (SUD) in fifty cases. *Current Psychiatry Research and Reviews.*

13. Melnick, M. (Dec. 4, 2014). Turns out, your vegetarianism probably is just a phase. *HuffPost.*

14. Ocean, N., Howley, P., & Ensor, J. (2019). Lettuce be happy: a longitudinal UK study on the relationship between fruit and vegetable consumption and well-being. *Social Science & Medicine.*

15. Teicholz, N. (2014). *The Big Fat Surprise.*

16. Guasch-Ferré, M., & Willett, W. C. (2021). The Mediterranean diet and health: a comprehensive overview. *Journal of Internal Medicine.*

17. Martínez-González, M. A., & Gea, A. (2012). Mediterranean diet: the whole is more than the sum of its parts. *British Journal of Nutrition.*

18. Thomsen, S. T., de Boer, W., Pires, S. M., Devleesschauwer, B., Fagt, S., Andersen, R., Poulsen, M., & van der Voet, H. (2019). A probabilistic approach for risk-benefit assessment of food substitutions: a case study on substituting meat by fish. *Food and Chemical Toxicology.*

19. Darmadi-Blackberry, I., Wahlqvist, M. L., Kouris-Blazos, A., Steen, B., Lukito, W., Horie, Y., & Horie, K. (2004). Legumes: the most important dietary predictor of survival in older people of different ethnicities. *Asia Pacific Journal of Clinical Nutrition.*

20. Bassett, D. R., Jr, Wyatt, H. R., Thompson, H., Peters, J. C., & Hill, J. O. (2010). Pedometer-measured physical activity and health behaviors in U.S. adults. *Medicine and Science in Sports and Exercise.*

21. Paluch, A., Gabriel, K., Fulton, J., Lewis, C., Schreiner, P., Sternfeld, B., Sidney, S., Siddique, J., Whitaker, K., Carnethon, M., (2021). Steps per day and all-cause mortality in middle-aged adults in the Coronary Artery Risk Development in Young Adults study. *JAMA Network Open.*

22. Lee, I., Shiroma, E., & Kamada, M., (2019). Association of step volume and intensity with all-cause mortality in older women. *JAMA Internal Medicine.*

23. Del Pozo Cruz, B., Ahmadi, M. N., Lee, I. M., & Stamatakis, E. (2022). Prospective associations of daily step counts and intensity with cancer and cardiovascular disease incidence and mortality and all-cause mortality. *JAMA Internal Medicine.*

24. Del Pozo Cruz, B., Ahmadi, M., Naismith, S. L., & Stamatakis, E. (2022). Association of daily step count and intensity with incident dementia in 78,430 adults living in the UK. *JAMA Neurology.*

25. Blackwell, D. L., & Clarke, T. C. (2018). State variation in meeting the 2008 federal guidelines for both aerobic and muscle-strengthening activities through leisure-time physical activity among adults aged 18-64: United States, 2010–2015. *National Health Statistics Reports.*

26. Cochrane, M. (March 15, 2012). No major change in Americans' exercise habits in 2011. *Gallup.com.*

27. Kohyama J. (2021). Which is more important for health: sleep quantity or sleep quality? *Children.*

28. Gringras, P., Middleton, B., Skene, D. J., & Revell, V. L. (2015). Bigger, brighter, bluer–better? Current light-emitting devices: adverse sleep properties and preventative strategies. *Frontiers in Public Health*.

29. Khubchandani, J., Price, J. H., Sharma, S., Wiblishauser, M. J., & Webb, F. J. (2022). COVID-19 pandemic and weight gain in American adults: a nationwide population-based study. *Diabetes & Metabolic Syndrome*.

30. Tison, G. H., Barrios, J., Avram, R., Kuhar, P., Bostjancic, B., Marcus, G. M., Pletcher, M. J., & Olgin, J. E. (2022). Worldwide physical activity trends since COVID-19 onset. *Lancet*.

31. Ingraham, C. (Oct. 30, 2019). Actually, you do have enough time to exercise, and here's the data to prove it. *Washington Post*.

Chapter 3

1. Mead, S., & Knott, M. (1966). Topical cryotherapy-use for relief of pain and spasticity. *California Medicine*.

2. Radecka, A., Knyszyńska, A., Łuczak, J., & Lubkowska, A. (2021). Adaptive changes in muscle activity after cryotherapy treatment: potential mechanism for improvement of the functional state in patients with multiple sclerosis. *NeuroRehabilitation*.

3. Pawik, M., Kowalska, J., & Rymaszewska, J. (2019). The effectiveness of whole-body cryotherapy and physical exercises on the psychological well-being of patients with multiple sclerosis: a comparative analysis. *Advances in Clinical and Experimental Medicine*.

4. Lateef F. (2010). Post exercise ice water immersion: is it a form of active recovery? *Journal of Emergencies, Trauma, and Shock*.

5. Cuce, S. (Feb. 8, 2012). The Dallas Mavericks' "secret weapon": cryotherapy. *Deadspin*.

6. Boyles, S. (Oct. 16, 2008). Phiten necklace: baseball boost or myth? *CBSnews.com*.

7. Hausswirth, C., Louis, J., Bieuzen, F., Pournot, H., Fournier, J., Filliard, J. R., & Brisswalter, J. (2011). Effects of whole-body cryotherapy vs. far-infrared vs. passive modalities on recovery from exercise-induced muscle damage in highly-trained runners. *PloS One*.

8. Ziemann, E., Olek, R. A., Kujach, S., Grzywacz, T., Antosiewicz, J., Garsztka, T., & Laskowski, R. (2012). Five-day whole-body cryostimulation, blood inflammatory markers, and performance in high-ranking professional tennis players. *Journal of Athletic Training*.

9. Mila-Kierzenkowska, C., Jurecka, A., Woźniak, A., Szpinda, M., Augustyńska, B., & Woźniak, B. (2013). The effect of submaximal exercise preceded by single whole-body cryotherapy on the markers of oxidative stress and inflammation in blood of volleyball players. *Oxidative Medicine and Cellular Longevity*.

10. Ziemann, E., Olek, R. A., Grzywacz, T., Kaczor, J. J., Antosiewicz, J., Skrobot, W., Kujach, S., & Laskowski, R. (2014). Whole-body cryostimulation as an effective way of reducing exercise-induced inflammation and blood cholesterol in young men. *European Cytokine Network*.

11. Bouzigon, R., Dupuy, O., Tiemessen, I., De Nardi, M., Bernard, J. P., Mihailovic, T., Theurot, D., Miller, E. D., Lombardi, G., & Dugué, B. M. (2021). Cryostimulation for post-exercise recovery in athletes: a consensus and position paper. *Frontiers in Sports and Active Living*.

12. Rodriguez-Pintó, I., Agmon-Levin, N., Howard, A., & Shoenfeld, Y. (2014). Fibromyalgia and cytokines. *Immunology Letters*.

13. Klemm, P., Becker, J., Aykara, I., Asendorf, T., Dischereit, G., Neumann, E., Müller-Ladner, U., & Lange, U. (2021). Serial whole-body cryotherapy in fibromyalgia is effective and alters cytokine profiles. *Advances in Rheumatology*.

14. Yilmaz, N., & Kiyak, E. (2017). The effects of local cold application on fibromyalgia pain. *International Journal of Rheumatic Diseases*.

15. Nelson, S. (Dec 2, 2021). Could cryotherapy help your eczema? *National eczema.org*.

16. Fischer, A. H., Shin, D. B., Margolis, D. J., & Takeshita, J. (2017). Racial and ethnic differences in health care utilization for childhood eczema: an analysis of the 2001–2013 Medical Expenditure Panel Surveys. *Journal of the American Academy of Dermatology*.

17. Wan, J., Margolis, D. J., Mitra, N., Hoffstad, O. J., & Takeshita, J. (2019). Racial and ethnic differences in atopic dermatitis-related school absences among US children. *JAMA Dermatology*.

18. Nutten S. (2015). Atopic dermatitis: global epidemiology and risk factors. *Annals of Nutrition & Metabolism*.

19. eHealth (2020). ACA Index Report on Unsubsidized Consumers in the 2020 Open Enrollment Period.

20. Simpson, E. L., Bieber, T., Guttman-Yassky, E., Beck, L. A., Blauvelt, A., Cork, M. J., Silverberg, J. I., Deleuran, M., Kataoka, Y., Lacour, J. P., Kingo, K., Worm, M., Poulin, Y., Wollenberg, A., Soo, Y., Graham, N. M., Pirozzi,

G., Akinlade, B., Staudinger, H., Mastey, V., Eckert, L., Gadkari, A., Stahl, N., Yancopoulos, G., Ardeleanu, M., SOLO 1 and SOLO 2 Investigators (2016). Two phase 3 trials of Dupilumab versus placebo in atopic dermatitis. *New England Journal of Medicine.*

21. Klimenko, T., Ahvenainen, S., & Karvonen, S. L. (2008). Whole-body cryotherapy in atopic dermatitis. *Archives of Dermatology.*

22. Lee, E. H., Lee, H. J., Park, K. D., & Lee, W. J. (2021). Effect of a new cryotherapy device on an itchy sensation in patients with mild atopic dermatitis. *Journal of Cosmetic Dermatology.*

23. Kepinska-Szyszkowska, M., Misiorek, A., Kapinska-Mrowiecka, M., Tabak, J., & Malina, K. (2020). Assessment of the influence systemic cryotherapy exerts on chosen skin scores of patients with atopic dermatitis: pilot study. *Biomed Research International.*

24. Rymaszewska, J., Tulczynski, A., Zagrobelny, Z., Kiejna, A., & Hadrys, T. (2003). Influence of whole body cryotherapy on depressive symptoms - preliminary report. *Acta Neuropsychiatrica.*

25. Pawik, M., Kowalska, J., & Rymaszewska, J. (2019). The effectiveness of whole-body cryotherapy and physical exercises on the psychological well-being of patients with multiple sclerosis: a comparative analysis. *Advances in Clinical and Experimental Medicine.*

26. Rymaszewska, J., Lion, K. M., Pawlik-Sobecka, L., Pawłowski, T., Szcześniak, D., Trypka, E., Rymaszewska, J. E., Zabłocka, A., & Stanczykiewicz, B. (2020). Efficacy of the whole-body cryotherapy as add-on therapy to pharmacological treatment of depression: a randomized controlled trial. *Frontiers in Psychiatry.*

27. Senczyszyn, A., Wallner, R., Szczesniak, D. M., Łuc, M., & Rymaszewska, J. (2021). The effectiveness of computerized cognitive training combined with whole body cryotherapy in improving cognitive functions in older adults: a case control study. *Frontiers in Psychiatry.*

28. Theurot, D., Dugué, B., Douzi, W., Guitet, P., Louis, J., & Dupuy, O. (2021). Impact of acute partial-body cryostimulation on cognitive performance, cerebral oxygenation, and cardiac autonomic activity. *Scientific Reports.*

29. David, A. (April 22, 2016). I tried cryotherapy as a treatment for depression. *Psychology Today.*

30. Mumby, H. S., Courtiol, A., Mar, K. U., & Lummaa, V. (2013). Climatic variation and age-specific survival in Asian elephants from Myanmar. *Ecology.*

31. Gribble, K. E., Moran, B. M., Jones, S., Corey, E. L., & Mark Welch, D. B.

(2018). Congeneric variability in lifespan extension and onset of senescence suggest active regulation of aging in response to low temperature. *Experimental Gerontology.*

32. Coolbaugh, C. L., Damon, B. M., Bush, E. C., Welch, E. B., & Towse, T. F. (2019). Cold exposure induces dynamic, heterogeneous alterations in human brown adipose tissue lipid content. *Scientific Reports.*

33. Sinclar, D. & LaPlante, M. (2019). *Lifespan: Why We Age and Why We Don't Have To.*

34. Buijze, G. A., Sierevelt, I. N., van der Heijden, B. C., Dijkgraaf, M. G., & Frings-Dresen, M. H. (2016). The effect of cold showering on health and work: a randomized controlled trial. *PloS One.*

35. Srámek, P., Simecková, M., Janský, L., Savlíková, J., & Vybíral, S. (2000). Human physiological responses to immersion into water of different temperatures. *European Journal of Applied Physiology.*

Chapter 4

1. Davis-Flynn, J. (July 23, 2021). I used an infrared sauna for 30 days—here's what happened. *Yoga Journal.*

2. Adams, F. (1834). *The Medical Works of Paulus Aegineta.*

3. Brunt, V. E., & Minson, C. T. (2021). Heat therapy: mechanistic underpinnings and applications to cardiovascular health. *Journal of Applied Physiology.*

4. Laukkanen, T., Khan, H., Zaccardi, F., & Laukkanen, J. A. (2015). Association between sauna bathing and fatal cardiovascular and all-cause mortality events. *JAMA Internal Medicine.*

5. Laukkanen, T., Kunutsor, S. K., Khan, H., Willeit, P., Zaccardi, F., & Laukkanen, J. A. (2018). Sauna bathing is associated with reduced cardiovascular mortality and improves risk prediction in men and women: a prospective cohort study. *BMC Medicine.*

6. Nakamura, M., Sugawara, S., Arakawa, N., Nagano, M., Shizuka, T., Shimoda, Y., Sakai, T., & Hiramori, K. (2004). Reduced vascular compliance is associated with impaired endothelium-dependent dilatation in the brachial artery of patients with congestive heart failure. *Journal of Cardiac Failure.*

7. Laatikainen, T., Salminen, K., Kohvakka, A., & Pettersson, J. (1988). Response of plasma endorphins, prolactin and catecholamines in women to intense heat in a sauna. *European Journal of Applied Physiology and Occupational Physiology.*

8. Huhtaniemi, I., & Laukkanen, J. (2020). Endocrine effects of sauna bath. *Current Opinion in Endocrine and Metabolic Research.*

9. Laukkanen, T., Laukkanen, J. A., & Kunutsor, S. K. (2018). Sauna bathing and risk of psychotic disorders: A prospective cohort study. *Medical Principles and Practice.*

10. Richmond-Rakerd, L. S., D'Souza, S., Milne, B. J., Caspi, A., & Moffitt, T. E. (2022). Longitudinal associations of mental disorders with dementia: 30-year analysis of 1.7 million New Zealand citizens. *JAMA Psychiatry.*

11. Laukkanen, T., Kunutsor, S., Kauhanen, J., & Laukkanen, J. A. (2017). Sauna bathing is inversely associated with dementia and Alzheimer's disease in middle-aged Finnish men. *Age and Ageing.*

12. Shinsato, T., Miyata, M., Kubozono, T., Ikeda, Y., Fujita, S., Kuwahata, S., Akasaki, Y., Hamasaki, S., Fujiwara, H., & Tei, C. (2010). Waon therapy mobilizes CD34+ cells and improves peripheral arterial disease. *Journal of Cardiology.*

13. Oosterveld, F. G., Rasker, J. J., Floors, M., Landkroon, R., van Rennes, B., Zwijnenberg, J., van de Laar, M. A., & Koel, G. J. (2009). Infrared sauna in patients with rheumatoid arthritis and ankylosing spondylitis: a pilot study showing good tolerance, short-term improvement of pain and stiffness, and a trend towards long-term beneficial effects. *Clinical Rheumatology.*

14. Nurmikko, T., & Hietaharju, A. (1992). Effect of exposure to sauna heat on neuropathic and rheumatoid pain. *Pain.*

15. Chacko, S. M., Thambi, P. T., Kuttan, R., & Nishigaki, I. (2010). Beneficial effects of green tea: a literature review. *Chinese Medicine.*

16. Hayasaka, S., Goto, Y., & Maeda-Yamamoto, M. (2013). The effects of bathing in hot springs on the absorption of green tea catechin: a pilot study. *Complementary Therapies in Clinical Practice.*

17. Laukkanen, J. A., Laukkanen, T., & Kunutsor, S. K. (2018). Cardiovascular and other health benefits of sauna bathing: a review of the evidence. *Mayo Clinic Proceedings.*

18. Patrick, R. P., & Johnson, T. L. (2021). Sauna use as a lifestyle practice to extend healthspan. *Experimental Gerontology.*

19. Shadgan, B., Pakravan, A. H., Hoens, A., & Reid, W. D. (2018). Contrast baths, intramuscular hemodynamics, and oxygenation as monitored by near-infrared spectroscopy. *Journal of Athletic Training.*

20. Bieuzen, F., Bleakley, C. M., & Costello, J. T. (2013). Contrast water therapy and exercise induced muscle damage: a systematic review and meta-analysis. *PloS One.*

21. Sinclair, D. A., & LaPlante, M. D. (2019). *Lifespan: Why We Age—and Why We Don't Have To.*

22. Laukkanen, T., Kunutsor, S., Kauhanen, J., & Laukkanen, J. A. (2017). Sauna bathing is inversely associated with dementia and Alzheimer's disease in middle-aged Finnish men. *Age and Ageing.*

23. Kunutsor, S. K., Laukkanen, T., & Laukkanen, J. A. (2017). Frequent sauna bathing may reduce the risk of pneumonia in middle-aged Caucasian men: the KIHD prospective cohort study. *Respiratory Medicine.*

24. Kunutsor, S. K., Laukkanen, T., & Laukkanen, J. A. (2017). Sauna bathing reduces the risk of respiratory diseases: a long-term prospective cohort study. *European Journal of Epidemiology.*

25. Kunutsor, S. K., Khan, H., Zaccardi, F., Laukkanen, T., Willeit, P., & Laukkanen, J. A. (2018). Sauna bathing reduces the risk of stroke in Finnish men and women: a prospective cohort study. *Neurology.*

26. Kunutsor, S. K., Laukkanen, T., & Laukkanen, J. A. (2018). Longitudinal associations of sauna bathing with inflammation and oxidative stress: the KIHD prospective cohort study. *Annals of Medicine.*

27. Laukkanen, J. A., Mäkikallio, T. H., Khan, H., Laukkanen, T., Kauhanen, J., & Kunutsor, S. K. (2019). Finnish sauna bathing does not increase or decrease the risk of cancer in men: a prospective cohort study. *European Journal of Cancer.*

Chapter 5

1. Park, H. Y., Park, W., & Lim, K. (2019). Living high-training low for 21 days enhances exercise economy, hemodynamic function, and exercise performance of competitive runners. *Journal of Sports Science & Medicine.*

2. Kramnick, I. (1986). Eighteenth-century science and radical social theory: the case of Joseph Priestley's scientific liberalism. *Journal of British Studies.*

3. Krishnamurti, C. (2019). Historical aspects of hyperbaric physiology and medicine. *Respiratory Physiology.*

4. Brummelkamp, W., Hogendijk, L., & Boerema, I. (1961). Treatment of anaerobic infections (Clostridial myositis) by drenching the tissues with oxygen under high atmospheric pressure. *Surgery.*

5. Smith, G. & Sharp, G. (1960). Treatment of carbon-monoxide poisoning with oxygen under pressure. *Lancet.*

6. Perrins, J., Maudsley, R., Colwill, M., & Slack, W. (1966). Thomas DAOHP

in the management of chronic osteomyelitis. *Proceedings of the Third International Conference on Hyperbaric Medicine.*

7. Saltzman, H., Heyman, A., & Whalen, R. (1966). The use of hyperbaric oxygen in the treatment of cerebral ischemia and infarction. *Circulation.*

8. Thurston, G., Greenwood, T., Bending, M., Connor, H., & Curwen, M. (1973). A controlled investigation into the effects of hyperbaric oxygen on mortality following acute myocardial infarction. *Quarterly Journal of Medicine.*

9. Neubauer, R., Gottlieb, S., & Kagan, R. (1990). Enhancing "idling" neurons. *Lancet.*

10. Marx, R., Johnson, R., & Kline, S. (1985). Prevention of osteoradionecrosis: a randomized prospective clinical trial of hyperbaric oxygen versus penicillin. *Journal of the American Dental Association.*

11. Hood, L. & Price, N. (2023). *The Age of Scientific Wellness: Why the Future of Medicine Is Personalized, Predictive, Data-Rich, and in Your Hands.*

12. Sheffield, P. J., & Desautels, D. A. (1997). Hyperbaric and hypobaric chamber fires: a 73-year analysis. *Undersea & Hyperbaric Medicine.*

13. The Vitality Health Show (Feb. 10, 2022).

14. Holland H. D. (2006). The oxygenation of the atmosphere and oceans. *Philosophical Transactions of the Royal Society of London. Series B, Biological Sciences.*

15. Zhang, H., Zang, C., Xu, Z., Zhang, Y., Xu, J., Bian, J., Morozyuk, D., Khullar, D., Zhang, Y., Nordvig, A. S., Schenck, E. J., Shenkman, E. A., Rothman, R. L., Block, J. P., Lyman, K., Weiner, M. G., Carton, T. W., Wang, F., & Kaushal, R. (2023). Data-driven identification of post-acute SARS-CoV-2 infection subphenotypes. *Nature Medicine.*

16. Robbins, T., Gonevski, M., Clark, C., Baitule, S., Sharma, K., Magar, A., Patel, K., Sankar, S., Kyrou, I., Ali, A., & Randeva, H. S. (2021). Hyperbaric oxygen therapy for the treatment of long COVID: early evaluation of a highly promising intervention. *Clinical Medicine.*

17. El Hawa, A. A. A., Charipova, K., Bekeny, J. C., & Johnson-Arbor, K. K. (2021). The evolving use of hyperbaric oxygen therapy during the COVID-19 pandemic. *Journal of Wound Care.*

18. Kious, B. M., Kondo, D. G., & Renshaw, P. F. (2018). Living high and feeling low: altitude, suicide, and depression. *Harvard Review of Psychiatry.*

19. Kious, B. M., Bakian, A., Zhao, J., Mickey, B., Guille, C., Renshaw, P., & Sen,

S. (2019). Altitude and risk of depression and anxiety: findings from the intern health study. *International Review of Psychiatry.*

20. Østergaard, L., Jørgensen, M. B., & Knudsen, G. M. (2018). Low on energy? An energy supply-demand perspective on stress and depression. *Neuroscience and Biobehavioral Reviews.*

21. Canadian Agency for Drugs and Technologies in Health. (2014). Hyperbaric oxygen therapy for adults with mental illness: a review of the clinical effectiveness.

22. Cao, H., Ju, K., Zhong, L., & Meng, T. (2013). Efficacy of hyperbaric oxygen treatment for depression in the convalescent stage following cerebral hemorrhage. *Experimental and Therapeutic Medicine.*

23. Yan, D., Shan, J., Ze, Y., Xiao-Yan, Z., & Xiao-Hua, H. (2015). The effects of combined hyperbaric oxygen therapy on patients with post-stroke depression. *Journal of Physical Therapy Science.*

24. Feng, J. J., & Li, Y. H. (2017). Effects of hyperbaric oxygen therapy on depression and anxiety in the patients with incomplete spinal cord injury. *Medicine.*

25. Bloch, Y., Belmaker, R. H., Shvartzman, P., Romem, P., Bolotin, A., Bersudsky, Y., & Azab, A. N. (2021). Normobaric oxygen treatment for mild-to-moderate depression: a randomized, double-blind, proof-of-concept trial. *Scientific Reports.*

26. Institute for Quality and Efficiency in Health Care. (2006). Depression: how effective are antidepressants?

27. Almohammed, O. A., Alsalem, A. A., Almangour, A. A., Alotaibi, L. H., Al Yami, M. S., & Lai, L. (2022). Antidepressants and health-related quality of life (HRQoL) for patients with depression: analysis of the medical expenditure panel survey from the United States. *PloS One.*

28. Wenner Moyer, M. (April 21, 2022). How much do antidepressants help, really? *New York Times.*

29. Schottlender, N., Gottfried, I., & Ashery, U. (2021). Hyperbaric oxygen treatment: effects on mitochondrial function and oxidative stress. *Biomolecules.*

30. Hadanny, A., & Efrati, S. (2020). The hyperoxic-hypoxic paradox. *Biomolecules.*

31. Ding, J., Zhou, D., Liu, C., Pan, L., Ya, J., Ding, Y., Ji, X., & Meng, R. (2019). Normobaric oxygen: a novel approach for treating chronic cerebral circulation insufficiency. *Clinical Interventions in Aging.*

32. Ding, J., Liu, Y., Li, X., Chen, Z., Guan, J., Jin, K., Wang, Z., Ding, Y., Ji, X., & Meng, R. (2020). Normobaric oxygen may ameliorate cerebral venous outflow disturbance-related neurological symptoms. *Frontiers in Neurology.*

33. Mendham, A. E., Goedecke, J. H., Zeng, Y., Larsen, S., George, C., Hauksson, J., Fortuin-de Smidt, M. C., Chibalin, A. V., Olsson, T., & Chorell, E. (2021). Exercise training improves mitochondrial respiration and is associated with an altered intramuscular phospholipid signature in women with obesity. *Diabetologia*.

34. Sorriento, D., Di Vaia, E., & Iaccarino, G. (2021). Physical exercise: a novel tool to protect mitochondrial health. *Frontiers in Physiology*.

35. Burtscher M. (2020). A breath of fresh air for mitochondria in exercise physiology. *Acta Physiologica*.

36. Luttmann-Gibson, H., Sarnat, S. E., Suh, H. H., Coull, B. A., Schwartz, J., Zanobetti, A., & Gold, D. R. (2014). Short-term effects of air pollution on oxygen saturation in a cohort of senior adults in Steubenville, Ohio. *Journal of Occupational and Environmental Medicine*.

37. Han, K. T., & Ruan, L. W. (2020). Effects of indoor plants on air quality: a systematic review. *Environmental Science and Pollution Research International*.

38. Mayer, A. F., Karloh, M., Dos Santos, K., de Araujo, C. L. P., & Gulart, A. A. (2018). Effects of acute use of pursed-lips breathing during exercise in patients with COPD: a systematic review and meta-analysis. *Physiotherapy*.

Chapter 6

1. Bear, T., Philipp, M., Hill, S., & Mündel, T. (2016). A preliminary study on how hypohydration affects pain perception. *Psychophysiology*.

2. Wu, Q., & Huang, J. H. (2017). Intervertebral disc aging, degeneration, and associated potential molecular mechanisms. *Journal of Head, Neck & Spine Surgery*.

3. Watson, P. E., Watson, I. D., & Batt, R. D. (1980). Total body water volumes for adult males and females estimated from simple anthropometric measurements. *American Journal of Clinical Nutrition*.

4. Barley, O. R., Chapman, D. W., & Abbiss, C. R. (2020). Reviewing the current methods of assessing hydration in athletes. *Journal of the International Society of Sports Nutrition*.

5. Goodman, A. B., Blanck, H. M., Sherry, B., Park, S., Nebeling, L., & Yaroch, A. L. (2013). Behaviors and attitudes associated with low drinking water intake among US adults, food attitudes and behaviors survey, 2007. *Preventing Chronic Disease*.

6. Weinberg, A. D., & Minaker, K. L. (1995). Dehydration. Evaluation and management in older adults. *JAMA*.

7. Amiri, P., Kazeminasab, S., Nejadghaderi, S. A., Mohammadinasab, R., Pourfathi, H., Araj-Khodaei, M., Sullman, M. J. M., Kolahi, A. A., & Safiri,

S. (2022). Migraine: a review on its history, global epidemiology, risk factors, and comorbidities. *Frontiers in Neurology.*

8. Bron, C., Sutherland, H. G., & Griffiths, L. R. (2021). Exploring the hereditary nature of migraine. *Neuropsychiatric Disease and Treatment.*

9. Khorsha, F., Mirzababaei, A., Togha, M., & Mirzaei, K. (2020). Association of drinking water and migraine headache severity. *Journal of Clinical Neuroscience.*

10. Arca, K. N., & Halker Singh, R. B. (2021). Dehydration and headache. *Current Pain and Headache Reports.*

11. Duning, T., Kloska, S., Steinsträter, O., Kugel, H., Heindel, W., & Knecht, S. (2005). Dehydration confounds the assessment of brain atrophy. *Neurology.*

12. McCotter, L., Douglas, P., Laur, C., Gandy, J., Fitzpatrick, L., Rajput-Ray, M., & Ray, S. (2016). Hydration education: developing, piloting and evaluating a hydration education package for general practitioners. *BMJ Open.*

13. Nowaczewska, M., Wiciński, M., & Kaźmierczak, W. (2020). The ambiguous role of caffeine in migraine headache: From trigger to treatment. *Nutrients.*

14. Gelfand, A. A., & Goadsby, P. J. (2012). A neurologist's guide to acute migraine therapy in the emergency room. *Neurohospitalist.*

15. Chuda, A., Kaszkowiak, M., Banach, M., Maciejewski, M., & Bielecka-Dabrowa, A. (2021). The relationship of dehydration and body mass index with the occurrence of atrial fibrillation in heart failure patients. *Frontiers in Cardiovascular Medicine.*

16. Day, J. D., Bunch. T. J., & LaPlante, M. D. (2021). *The AFib Cure: Get Off Your Medications, Take Control of Your Health, and Add Years to Your Life.*

17. Cacioppo, F., Reisenbauer, D., Herkner, H., Oppenauer, J., Schuetz, N., Niederdoeckl, J., Schnaubelt, S., Gupta, S., Lutnik, M., Simon, A., Spiel, A. O., Buchtele, N., Domanovits, H., Laggner, A. N., & Schwameis, M. (2022). Association of intravenous potassium and magnesium administration with spontaneous conversion of atrial fibrillation and atrial flutter in the emergency department. *JAMA Network Open.*

18. Zhang, J., Zhang, N., Du, S., He, H., Xu, Y., Cai, H., Guo, X., & Ma, G. (2018). The effects of hydration status on cognitive performances among young adults in Hebei, China: A randomized controlled trial. *International Journal of Environmental Research and Public Health.*

19. Zhang, J., Ma, G., Du, S., Liu, S., & Zhang, N. (2021). Effects of water restriction and supplementation on cognitive performances and mood among young adults in Baoding, China: A randomized controlled trial. *Nutrients.*

20. Zhang, N., Zhang, J., Du, S., & Ma, G. (2022). Dehydration and rehydration affect brain regional density and homogeneity among young male adults, determined via magnetic resonance imaging: A pilot self-control trial. *Frontiers in Nutrition.*

21. Stare, F. & McWilliams, M. (1974). *Nutrition for Good Health.*

22. Valtin H. (2002). "Drink at least eight glasses of water a day." Really? Is there scientific evidence for '8 x 8'? *American Journal of Physiology: Regulatory, Integrative and Comparative Physiology.*

23. Popkin, B. M., D'Anci, K. E., & Rosenberg, I. H. (2010). Water, hydration, and health. *Nutrition Reviews.*

Chapter 7

1. Dean, J. (March 15, 2022). A third of U.S. adults are struggling to get a good night's rest, a survey finds. *NPR.org.*

2. Clark-Flory, T. (July 3, 2021). What's better than sex? *Salon.*

3. Counting Sheep Podcast. https://soundcloud.com/user-667883117.

4. Lauderdale, D. S., Knutson, K. L., Yan, L. L., Liu, K., & Rathouz, P. J. (2008). Self-reported and measured sleep duration: How similar are they? *Epidemiology.*

5. Ekirch A. R. (2016). Segmented sleep in preindustrial societies. *Sleep.*

6. Hussain, J. N., Greaves, R. F., & Cohen, M. M. (2019). A hot topic for health: results of the Global Sauna Survey. *Complementary Therapies in Medicine.*

7. Jayson, J., Montgomery, I., & Trinder, J. (1990). The effect of afternoon body heating on body temperature and slow wave sleep. *Psychophysiology.*

8. Stutz, J., Eiholzer, R., & Spengler, C. M. (2019). Effects of evening exercise on sleep in healthy participants: a systematic review and meta-analysis. *Sports Medicine.*

9. Jehan, S., Zizi, F., Pandi-Perumal, S. R., Wall, S., Auguste, E., Myers, A. K., Jean-Louis, G., & McFarlane, S. I. (2017). Obstructive sleep apnea and obesity: implications for public health. *Sleep Medicine and Disorders.*

10. Goldman, S. E., Hall, M., Boudreau, R., Matthews, K. A., Cauley, J. A., Ancoli-Israel, S., Stone, K. L., Rubin, S. M., Satterfield, S., Simonsick, E. M., & Newman, A. B. (2008). Association between nighttime sleep and napping in older adults. *Sleep.*

11. Long, Y., Tan, J., Nie, Y., Lu, Y., Mei, X., & Tu, C. (2017). Hyperbaric oxygen therapy is safe and effective for the treatment of sleep disorders in children with cerebral palsy. *Neurological Research.*

12. Walker, J. M., Mulatya, C., Hebert, D., Wilson, S. H., Lindblad, A. S., &

Weaver, L. K. (2018). Sleep assessment in a randomized trial of hyperbaric oxygen in U.S. service members with post concussive mild traumatic brain injury compared to normal controls. *Sleep Medicine.*

13. Wang, J., Wang, C., Wu, X., Ma, T., & Guo, X. (2022). Effect of hyperbaric oxygen therapy on sleep quality, drug dosage, and nerve function in patients with sleep disorders after ischemic cerebral stroke. *Emergency Medicine International.*

14. Hauer, B. E., Negash, B., Chan, K., Vuong, W., Colbourne, F., Pagliardini, S., & Dickson, C. T. (2018). Hyperoxia enhances slow-wave forebrain states in urethane-anesthetized and naturally sleeping rats. *Journal of Neurophysiology.*

15. Uezato, A., Enomoto, M., Tamaoka, M., Hobo, M., Inukai, S., Hideshima, M., Miyazaki, Y., Nishikawa, T., & Yagishita, K. (2017). Shorter sleep onset latency in patients undergoing hyperbaric oxygen treatment. *Psychiatry and Clinical Neurosciences.*

16. Shechter, A., Kim, E. W., St-Onge, M. P., & Westwood, A. J. (2018). Blocking nocturnal blue light for insomnia: A randomized controlled trial. *Journal of Psychiatric Research.*

17. Cornelis, M. C., El-Sohemy, A., Kabagambe, E. K., & Campos, H. (2006). Coffee, CYP1A2 genotype, and risk of myocardial infarction. *JAMA.*

18. Anderson, B. O., Berdzuli, N., Ilbawi, A., Kestel, D., Kluge, H. P., Krech, R., Mikkelsen, B., Neufeld, M., Poznyak, V., Rekve, D., Slama, S., Tello, J., & Ferreira-Borges, C. (2023). Health and cancer risks associated with low levels of alcohol consumption. *Lancet Public Health.*

19. Liu, J., Wu, T., Liu, Q., Wu, S., & Chen, J. C. (2020). Air pollution exposure and adverse sleep health across the life course: a systematic review. *Environmental Pollution.*

20. Halperin D. (2014). Environmental noise and sleep disturbances: a threat to health? *Sleep Science.*

21. Yazdannik, A. R., Zareie, A., Hasanpour, M., & Kashefi, P. (2014). The effect of earplugs and eye mask on patients' perceived sleep quality in intensive care unit. *Iranian Journal of Nursing and Midwifery Research.*

Chapter 8

1. Perelman, J., Serranheira, F., Pita Barros, P., & Laires, P. (2021). Does working at home compromise mental health? A study on European mature adults in COVID times. *Journal of Occupational Health.*

2. Platts, K., Breckon, J., & Marshall, E. (2022). Enforced home-working under

lockdown and its impact on employee wellbeing: a cross-sectional study. *BMC Public Health.*

3. Erickson, M. (June 3, 2020). Setting your biological clock, reducing stress while sheltering in place. *Scope.*

4. Slominski, A. T., Zmijewski, M. A., Plonka, P. M., Szaflarski, J. P., & Paus, R. (2018). How UV light touches the brain and endocrine system through skin, and why. *Endocrinology.*

5. Elliot A. J. (2015). Color and psychological functioning: a review of theoretical and empirical work. *Frontiers in Psychology.*

6. Okasha A. (1999). Mental health in the Middle East: an Egyptian perspective. *Clinical Psychology Review.*

7. Geddes, L. (2019). *Chasing the Sun: How the Science of Sunlight Shapes Our Bodies and Minds.*

8. Liebert, A., & Kiat, H. (2021). The history of light therapy in hospital physiotherapy and medicine with emphasis on Australia: evolution into novel areas of practice. *Physiotherapy Theory and Practice.*

9. Hamblin M. R. (2019). Photobiomodulation for Alzheimer's disease: has the light dawned? *Photonics.*

10. Schiffer, F., Johnston, A. L., Ravichandran, C., Polcari, A., Teicher, M. H., Webb, R. H., & Hamblin, M. R. (2009). Psychological benefits 2 and 4 weeks after a single treatment with near infrared light to the forehead: a pilot study of 10 patients with major depression and anxiety. *Behavioral and Brain Functions.*

11. Cassano, P., Cusin, C., Mischoulon, D., Hamblin, M. R., De Taboada, L., Pisoni, A., Chang, T., Yeung, A., Ionescu, D. F., Petrie, S. R., Nierenberg, A. A., Fava, M., & Iosifescu, D. V. (2015). Near-infrared transcranial radiation for major depressive disorder: proof of concept study. *Psychiatry Journal..*

12. Hipskind, S. G., Grover, F. L., Jr, Fort, T. R., Helffenstein, D., Burke, T. J., Quint, S. A., Bussiere, G., Stone, M., & Hurtado, T. (2018). Pulsed transcranial red/near-infrared light therapy using light-emitting diodes improves cerebral blood flow and cognitive function in veterans with chronic traumatic brain injury: a case series. *Photomedicine and Laser Surgery.*

13. Moreira, M. S., Velasco, I. T., Ferreira, L. S., Ariga, S. K., Barbeiro, D. F., Meneguzzo, D. T., Abatepaulo, F., & Marques, M. M. (2009). Effect of phototherapy with low intensity laser on local and systemic immunomodulation following focal brain damage in rat. *Journal of Photochemistry and Photobiology, B, Biology.*

14. Postolache, T. T., Wadhawan, A., Can, A., Lowry, C. A., Woodbury, M., Makkar, H., Hoisington, A. J., Scott, A. J., Potocki, E., Benros, M. E., & Stiller, J. W. (2020). Inflammation in traumatic brain injury. *Journal of Alzheimer's Disease.*

15. Quirk, B. J., Torbey, M., Buchmann, E., Verma, S., & Whelan, H. T. (2012). Near-infrared photobiomodulation in an animal model of traumatic brain injury: improvements at the behavioral and biochemical levels. *Photomedicine and Laser Surgery.*

16. Kinney, J. W., Bemiller, S. M., Murtishaw, A. S., Leisgang, A. M., Salazar, A. M., & Lamb, B. T. (2018). Inflammation as a central mechanism in Alzheimer's disease. *Alzheimer's & Dementia.*

17. De Taboada, L., Yu, J., El-Amouri, S., Gattoni-Celli, S., Richieri, S., McCarthy, T., Streeter, J., & Kindy, M. S. (2011). Transcranial laser therapy attenuates amyloid-β peptide neuropathology in amyloid-β protein precursor transgenic mice. *Journal of Alzheimer's Disease.*

18. Singh, B., Parsaik, A. K., Mielke, M. M., Erwin, P. J., Knopman, D. S., Petersen, R. C., & Roberts, R. O. (2014). Association of Mediterranean diet with mild cognitive impairment and Alzheimer's disease: a systematic review and meta-analysis. *Journal of Alzheimer's Disease.*

19. Hill, N. L., Kolanowski, A. M., & Gill, D. J. (2011). Plasticity in early Alzheimer's disease: an opportunity for intervention. *Topics in Geriatric Rehabilitation.*

20. Willis, S. L., & Schaie, K. W. (2009). Cognitive training and plasticity: theoretical perspective and methodological consequences. *Restorative Neurology and Neuroscience.*

21. Meng, Q., Lin, M. S., & Tzeng, I. S. (2020). Relationship between exercise and Alzheimer's disease: a narrative literature review. *Frontiers in Neuroscience.*

22. Justice N. J. (2018). The relationship between stress and Alzheimer's disease. *Neurobiology of Stress.*

23. Wong, T., Hsu, L., & Liao, W. (2013). Phototherapy in psoriasis: a review of mechanisms of action. *Journal of Cutaneous Medicine and Surgery.*

24. Veleva, B. I., van Bezooijen, R. L., Chel, V. G. M., Numans, M. E., & Caljouw, M. A. A. (2018). Effect of ultraviolet light on mood, depressive disorders and well-being. *Photodermatology, Photoimmunology & Photomedicine.*

25. Zhang, P., & Wu, M. X. (2018). A clinical review of phototherapy for psoriasis. *Lasers in Medical Science.*

26. Borsky, P., Chmelarova, M., Fiala, Z., Hamakova, K., Palicka, V., Krejsek, J.,

Andrys, C., Kremlacek, J., Rehacek, V., Beranek, M., Malkova, A., Svadlakova, T., Holmannova, D., & Borska, L. (2021). Aging in psoriasis vulgaris: female patients are epigenetically older than healthy controls. *Immunity & Ageing.*

27. Al-Atif H. (2022). Collagen supplements for aging and wrinkles: a paradigm shift in the fields of dermatology and cosmetics. *Dermatology Practical & Conceptual.*

28. Wunsch, A., & Matuschka, K. (2014). A controlled trial to determine the efficacy of red and near-infrared light treatment in patient satisfaction, reduction of fine lines, wrinkles, skin roughness, and intradermal collagen density increase. *Photomedicine and Laser Surgery.*

29. Ferraresi, C., Huang, Y. Y., & Hamblin, M. R. (2016). Photobiomodulation in human muscle tissue: an advantage in sports performance? *Journal of Biophotonics.*

30. Ferraresi, C., Bertucci, D., Schiavinato, J., Reiff, R., Araújo, A., Panepucci, R., Matheucci, E., Jr, Cunha, A. F., Arakelian, V. M., Hamblin, M. R., Parizotto, N., & Bagnato, V. (2016). Effects of light-emitting diode therapy on muscle hypertrophy, gene expression, performance, damage, and delayed-onset muscle soreness: case-control study with a pair of identical twins. *American Journal of Physical Medicine & Rehabilitation.*

31. Lokeshwar, S. D., Patel, P., Fantus, R. J., Halpern, J., Chang, C., Kargi, A. Y., & Ramasamy, R. (2021). Decline in serum testosterone levels among adolescent and young adult men in the USA. *European Urology Focus.*

32. Zupin, L., Pascolo, L., Luppi, S., Ottaviani, G., Crovella, S., & Ricci, G. (2020). Photobiomodulation therapy for male infertility. *Lasers in Medical Science.*

33. Cassano, P., Dording, C., Thomas, G., Foster, S., Yeung, A., Uchida, M., Hamblin, M. R., Bui, E., Fava, M., Mischoulon, D., & Iosifescu, D. V. (2019). Effects of transcranial photobiomodulation with near-infrared light on sexual dysfunction. *Lasers in Surgery and Medicine.*

34. Wright, K. P., Jr, McHill, A. W., Birks, B. R., Griffin, B. R., Rusterholz, T., & Chinoy, E. D. (2013). Entrainment of the human circadian clock to the natural light-dark cycle. *Current Biology.*

Chapter 9

1. Mujcic, R., & J Oswald, A. (2016). Evolution of well-being and happiness after increases in consumption of fruit and vegetables. *American Journal of Public Health.*

2. Faruque, S., Tong, J., Lacmanovic, V., Agbonghae, C., Minaya, D. M., &

Czaja, K. (2019). The dose makes the poison: sugar and obesity in the United States—a review. *Polish Journal of Food and Nutrition Sciences.*

3. Sinclair, A., Saeedi, P., Kaundal, A., Karuranga, S., Malanda, B., & Williams, R. (2020). Diabetes and global ageing among 65–99-year-old adults: findings from the International Diabetes Federation Diabetes Atlas, 9th edition. *Diabetes Research and Clinical Practice.*

4. Mann, T. (2015). *Secrets from the Eating Lab: The Science of Weight Loss, the Myth of Willpower, and Why You Should Never Diet Again.*

5. Ravussin, E., Redman, L. M., Rochon, J., Das, S. K., Fontana, L., Kraus, W. E., Romashkan, S., Williamson, D. A., Meydani, S. N., Villareal, D. T., Smith, S. R., Stein, R. I., Scott, T. M., Stewart, T. M., Saltzman, E., Klein, S., Bhapkar, M., Martin, C. K., Gilhooly, C. H., Holloszy, J. O., … CALERIE Study Group (2015). A 2-year randomized controlled trial of human caloric restriction: feasibility and effects on predictors of health span and longevity. *Journals of Gerontology. Series A, Biological Sciences and Medical Sciences.*

6. Moon, S., Kang, J., Kim, S. H., Chung, H. S., Kim, Y. J., Yu, J. M., Cho, S. T., Oh, C. M., & Kim, T. (2020). Beneficial effects of time-restricted eating on metabolic diseases: a systemic review and meta-analysis. *Nutrients.*

7. Su, Z., Li, R., & Gai, Z. (2018). Intravenous and nebulized magnesium sulfate for treating acute asthma in children: a systematic review and meta-analysis. *Pediatric Emergency Care.*

8. Tanzilli, G., Truscelli, G., Arrivi, A., Carnevale, R., Placanica, A., Viceconte, N., Raparelli, V., Mele, R., Cammisotto, V., Nocella, C., Barillà, F., Lucisano, L., Pennacchi, M., Granatelli, A., Dominici, M., Basili, S., Gaudio, C., & Mangieri, E. (2019). Glutathione infusion before primary percutaneous coronary intervention: a randomized controlled pilot study. *BMJ Open.*

9. Garrison, S. R., Korownyk, C. S., Kolber, M. R., Allan, G. M., Musini, V. M., Sekhon, R. K., & Dugré, N. (2020). Magnesium for skeletal muscle cramps. *Cochrane Database of Systematic Reviews.*

10. Avgerinos, K. I., Chatzisotiriou, A., Haidich, A. B., Tsapas, A., & Lioutas, V. A. (2019). Intravenous magnesium sulfate in acute stroke. *Stroke.*

11. Mahmoodpoor, A., Hamishehkar, H., Shadvar, K., Ostadi, Z., Sanaie, S., Saghaleini, S. H., & Nader, N. D. (2019). The effect of intravenous selenium on oxidative stress in critically ill patients with acute respiratory distress syndrome. *Immunological Investigations.*

12. Jafarnejad, S., Boccardi, V., Hosseini, B., Taghizadeh, M., & Hamedifard, Z. (2018). A meta-analysis of randomized control trials: the impact of vitamin

C supplementation on serum CRP and serum hs-CRP concentrations. *Current Pharmaceutical Design.*

13. Suh, S. Y., Bae, W. K., Ahn, H. Y., Choi, S. E., Jung, G. C., & Yeom, C. H. (2012). Intravenous vitamin C administration reduces fatigue in office workers: a double-blind randomized controlled trial. *Nutrition Journal.*

14. Shmerling, R. (Nov. 3, 2020). Drip bar: should you get an IV on demand? *Harvard Health Blog.*

15. Krzywański, J., Mikulski, T., Pokrywka, A., Młyńczak, M., Krysztofiak, H., Frączek, B., & Ziemba, A. (2020). Vitamin B12 status and optimal range for hemoglobin formation in elite athletes. *Nutrients.*

16. Martens, P. J., Gysemans, C., Verstuyf, A., & Mathieu, A. C. (2020). Vitamin D's effect on immune function. *Nutrients.*

17. Forrest, K. Y., & Stuhldreher, W. L. (2011). Prevalence and correlates of vitamin D deficiency in US adults. *Nutrition Research.*

18. Gupta, N., Farooqui, K. J., Batra, C. M., Marwaha, R. K., & Mithal, A. (2017). Effect of oral versus intramuscular vitamin D replacement in apparently healthy adults with Vitamin D deficiency. *Indian Journal of Endocrinology and Metabolism.*

19. Gorman, S., Zafirau, M. Z., Lim, E. M., Clarke, M. W., Dhamrait, G., Fleury, N., Walsh, J. P., Kaufmann, M., Jones, G., & Lucas, R. M. (2017). High-dose intramuscular vitamin D provides long-lasting moderate increases in serum 25-hydroxyvitamin D levels and shorter-term changes in plasma calcium. *Journal of AOAC International.*

20. Choi, H. S., Chung, Y. S., Choi, Y. J., Seo, D. H., & Lim, S. K. (2016). Efficacy and safety of vitamin D3 B.O.N. intramuscular injection in Korean adults with vitamin D deficiency. *Osteoporosis and Sarcopenia.*

21. Silvagno, F., Vernone, A., & Pescarmona, G. P. (2020). The role of glutathione in protecting against the severe inflammatory response triggered by COVID-19. *Antioxidants.*

22. Weschawalit, S., Thongthip, S., Phutrakool, P., & Asawanonda, P. (2017). Glutathione and its antiaging and antimelanogenic effects. *Clinical, Cosmetic and Investigational Dermatology.*

23. Burhan, E., & Wijaya, I. (2023). The role of high dose vitamin D and glutathione supplementation in COVID-19 treatment: a case series. *Journal of Infection in Developing Countries.*

24. Iskusnykh, I. Y., Zakharova, A. A., & Pathak, D. (2022). Glutathione in brain disorders and aging. *Molecules.*

25. Cohen, P. A., Avula, B., Katragunta, K., Travis, J. C., & Khan, I. (2023). Presence and quantity of botanical ingredients with purported performance-enhancing properties in sports supplements. *JAMA Network Open*.

26. Dickinson, A., Boyon, N., & Shao, A. (2009). Physicians and nurses use and recommend dietary supplements: report of a survey. *Nutrition Journal*.

27. Soutschek, A., Ruff, C. C., Strombach, T., Kalenscher, T., & Tobler, P. N. (2016). Brain stimulation reveals crucial role of overcoming self-centeredness in self-control. *Science Advances*.

Chapter 10

1. Scoon, G. S., Hopkins, W. G., Mayhew, S., & Cotter, J. D. (2007). Effect of post-exercise sauna bathing on the endurance performance of competitive male runners. *Journal of Science and Medicine in Sport*.

2. Matthews, C. E., Carlson, S. A., Saint-Maurice, P. F., Patel, S., Salerno, E. A., Loftfield, E., Troiano, R. P., Fulton, J. E., Sampson, J. N., Tribby, C., Keadle, S. K., & Berrigan, D. (2021). Sedentary behavior in U.S. adults: fall 2019. *Medicine and Science in Sports and Exercise*.

3. Puig-Ribera, A., Bort-Roig, J., Giné-Garriga, M., González-Suárez, A. M., Martínez-Lemos, I., Fortuño, J., Martori, J. C., Muñoz-Ortiz, L., Milà, R., Gilson, N. D., & McKenna, J. (2017). Impact of a workplace "sit less, move more" program on efficiency-related outcomes of office employees. *BMC Public Health*.

4. Roberts, A. (Sept. 20, 2021). The best workout routine ever, according to science. *Men's Journal*.

5. MacClurg, M. (Oct. 20, 2022). The real reason golf has helped pro athletes in retirement. *Golf Digest*.

6. Robinson, M. M., O'Leary, M. F. N., Nair, K. S., & Mitra, M. S. (2021). Acute high-intensity interval exercise increases markers of mitochondrial biogenesis in sedentary young adults. *American Journal of Physiology-Endocrinology and Metabolism*.

7. Ghosh, S., Leng, S., Kibbe, D., & Barochia, A. V. (2020). High-intensity interval training attenuates systemic inflammation in individuals with type 2 diabetes. *Diabetes Research and Clinical Practice*.

8. Little, J. P., Gillen, J. B., Percival, M. E., Safdar, A., Tarnopolsky, M. A., & Gibala, M. J. (2011). Low-volume high-intensity interval training reduces hyperglycemia and increases muscle mitochondrial capacity in patients with type 2 diabetes. *Journal of Applied Physiology*.

9. Gupta, S. K., Sawhney, J. P. S., Rai, R., Kumar, R., Srivastava, P., & Gupta, A.

(2019). Effects of high-intensity interval training versus moderate-intensity continuous training on blood pressure in adults with prehypertension to established hypertension: a systematic review and meta-analysis of randomized controlled trials. *European Journal of Preventive Cardiology.*

10. Aschwanden, C. (2019) *Good to Go: What the Athlete in All of Us Can Learn from the Strange Science of Recovery.*

11. Nelson, N. L. (2013). Massage therapy for the management of delayed onset muscle soreness: a systematic review. *Journal of Athletic Training.*

12. Hilbert, K., Rindfleisch, T., & Farber, J. (2018). Effects of massage on delayed-onset muscle soreness, swelling, and recovery of muscle function. *Journal of Sports Science and Medicine.*

13. Jayaseelan, D. J., Egan, B., & Sibbritt, D. (2017). Effects of sports massage on recovery of skeletal muscle from strenuous exercise. *International Journal of Sports Medicine.*

14. Hohenauer, E., Taeymans, J., Baeyens, J.-P., Clarys, P., & Clijsen, R. (2019). The effectiveness of whole-body cryotherapy compared to passive modalities on recovery from exercise-induced muscle damage in physically active adults: a systematic review and meta-analysis. *Sports Medicine.*

15. Beever, T., Tan, J. Y., Lee, Y. S., & Lim, C. L. (2021). The effects of post-exercise infrared sauna bathing on recovery from running-induced muscle damage in men: a randomized controlled trial. *PloS One.*

16. Wilson, M. A., Ainsworth, B. E., & Ahn, S. (2020). Effects of infrared sauna on recovery in collegiate men's basketball players. *Journal of Strength and Conditioning Research.*

17. McDermott, B. P., Anderson, S. A., Armstrong, L. E., Casa, D. J., Cheuvront, S. N., Cooper, L., Kenney, W. L., O'Connor, F. G., & Roberts, W. O. (2017). National Athletic Trainers' Association position statement: fluid replacement for the physically active. *Journal of Athletic Training.*

18. Hamblin, M. R. (2017). Mechanisms and applications of the anti-inflammatory effects of photobiomodulation. *AIMS Biophysics.*

19. Wang, W., Liu, K., Ma, L., Zeng, J., Yang, C., & Xu, H. (2019). The anti-inflammatory effects of hyperbaric oxygen therapy on tendon healing in rats. *PloS One.*

20. Zwerling, J. (Jan. 29, 2014). LeBron James, Kevin Durant help spearhead NBA popularity of legs recovery system. *Bleacher Report.*

21. Born, D. P., Sperlich, B., Holmberg, H. C., & Bringard, A. (2013). The effect of knee compression sleeves on running mechanics and

performance in trained distance runners. *Journal of Strength and Conditioning Research.*

Chapter 11

1. Holt-Lunstad, J., Smith, T. B., Baker, M., Harris, T., & Stephenson, D. (2015). Loneliness and social isolation as risk factors for mortality: a meta-analytic review. *Perspectives on Psychological Science.*
2. Eisenberger, N. I. (2012). The pain of social disconnection: examining the shared neural underpinnings of physical and social pain. *Nature Reviews Neuroscience.*
3. Gellert, P., Ziegelmann, J. P., Warner, L. M., & Schwarzer, R. (2011). Physical activity intervention in older adults: does a participating partner make a difference? *European Journal of Ageing.*
4. Day, J. (2017) *The Longevity Plan.* Harper.
5. Liebert, A., Bicknell, B., Markman, W., & Kiat, H. (2020). A Potential role for photobiomodulation therapy in disease treatment and prevention in the era of COVID-19. *Aging and Disease.*
6. Fowler, J. H., & Christakis, N. A. (2008). Dynamic spread of happiness in a large social network: longitudinal analysis over 20 years in the Framingham Heart Study. *BMJ.*
7. Carter, C. S., & Porges, S. W. (2013). The biochemistry of love: an oxytocin hypothesis. *EMBO Reports.*
8. Kraft, H. (2020). *Deep Kindness.*
9. King, P. (2022). *The Art of Self-Awareness.*
10. Allen, J. (2022). *Find Your People.*
11. Guzmán, M. (2022). *I Never Thought of It That Way.*
12. Cook, G. (Oct. 22, 2013). Why we are wired to connect. *Scientific American.*
13. Lyons, M. (Oct. 7, 2021). How to job hunt (when you're already exhausted). *Harvard Business Review.*
14. Epstein, S. (Oct. 1, 2020). Grieving the end an unhappy marriage or toxic friendship. *Psychology Today.*

Chapter 12

1. Wang, L., Wang, N., Zhang, W., Cheng, X., Yan, Z., Shao, G., Wang, X., Wang, R., & Fu, C. (2022). Therapeutic peptides: current applications and future directions. *Signal Transduction and Targeted Therapy.*
2. Wiecek, M., Szymura, J., Sproull, J., & Szygula, Z. (2020). Whole-body cryotherapy is an effective method of reducing abdominal obesity in menopausal women with metabolic syndrome. *Journal of Clinical Medicine.*

Index

acute injury pain, xxi, 89
aging, xxi, 13–14, 32
    age vs., 9–13
    and cryotherapy, 71–74
    disease and pain with, 29–31
    and exercise recovery, 197
    genetic view of, 10–11
    guides for success in, 236–237
    and heat therapy, 90–92
    and hydration, 120, 120, 133
    and movement, 203–208
    muscle mass decline with, 27–28
    nutrient deficiencies with, 28–29, 185
air quality, 117, 151–152
alcohol, 151
Alzheimer's disease, xxi, 85, 93, 164–166, 193
anxiety, xxi, 64, 109–111, 153, 153, 162
Aschwanden, Christie, 208–209
asthma, xxi, 185–188
athletic performance, xxi, 97–99, 171–172, 191–192, 202–208
athletic recovery, 58–63, 210–212
atopic dermatitis, 65–68
atrial fibrillation, xxi, 126–129
Attia, Peter, 32

back pain, xxi, 13–14, 119–120, 229
balance, xvii, 10, 196

Berman, Marvin, 165
biomarkers, 19
Brady, Tom, 59–60
brain health, 85–86, 129–130, 163–166
breathing practices, 117–118
Bredesen, Dale, 165

caffeine, 125, 127, 128, 151
caloric restriction, 184–185
cancer, 30–31, 93–94
Carlson, Tucker, 173
Carnegie Foundation for the Advancement of Teaching, 7–8
cellular psychology, 114–118
Celsus, Aulus Cornelius, 80–81
Charaka, 157
chronic pain, xxi, 15–16, 26, 63–64, 79
cognitive health, xxi
    and cryotherapy, 64, 69–71
    and heat therapy, 84–87
    and hydration, 120, 129–130, 133
    and light, 163–166
Cohen, Deborah, 49
cold therapy, 53–55, 75–77, 75–77. *see also* cryotherapy
compression therapy, 21–22, 211–212
connection(s), xvii, 215–226
    improving, 217–220
    new, building, 220–222

connection(s) (*cont.*)
    strengthening, 224–225
    support of family, 36
    toxic, 222–224
    with yourself, 218–219
contrast therapy, 92–93
COVID-19 pandemic, 153, 218
cryotherapy (cold therapy), xiv–xv, 53–77.
   see also cold therapy
    assessing safety of, 230–232
    for athletic recovery, 58–63
    for chronic pain, 63–64
    contrasting heat therapy and, 92–93
    for exercise recovery, 58–63, 210
    to maximize mobility, 55–58
    measuring success of, 240–241
    for mental and cognitive health,
      69–71
    podcasts focused on, 144–145
    for skin health, 65–68
    and sleep quality, 146
    to slow aging, 71–74
    whole-body, xi–xiv, 57, 60–65, 67–70
Cuban, Mark, 60
Cunningham, Orval, 101

David, Anna, 70
Davis-Flynn, Jennifer, 79
dehydration, 121–122
depression, xxi, 34–35, 243
    during COVID-19 pandemic, 153
    and cryotherapy, 64, 70
    and oxygen, 109–114
Dickson, Alma, 8
diet(s), 37–41
disease
    with aging, 12
    and heat therapy, 93–94
    and light therapy, 158–159
    as obstacle to wellness, 29–31
    other disease caused by, 30
    as starting point for treatment, 6–9
DNA testing, 19

Doyle, Bryson, 65
Drager, Heinrich, 101
Dupixent, 66–67

eating habits, xvii. *see also* nourishment
    and aging, 11
    and diets vs. individual plans, 177–179
    immediate effects of, 180–181
    to improve wellness, 37–41
    and nutrient absorption, 28–29
eczema, 65–68
Ekirch, Roger, 139
emotional resilience, xxi, 16
endurance, xxii, 98
energy, xvii, 242–243
    connection for, 219, 221–222
    hydration for, 133
    from hyper wellness journey, 228
    and nourishment, 190
    nourishment for, 181, 181–182
    oxygen for, 99
energy loss, xxii, 13–14, 26–28
    with excess weight, 40
    and light therapy, 164
    and toxic connections, 222–224
epigenome, 19, 178
Erickson, Mandy, 153, 154
European Medicines Agency, 11
exercise, xvii, 34. *see also* movement
    and aging, 11
    for atrial fibrillation, 127–129
    to counteract muscle mass decline, 27–28
    as hormetic stressor, 92
    to improve wellness, 41–44
    to increase oxygen flow, 117
    nourishment for, 181
    during pandemic, 49
    preparing muscles for, 55–57
    saunas before, 85
    and sleep, 142, 146–147
exercise recovery, xi–xiii, xxii, 21–22
    and cryotherapy, 58–63, 58–63
    and heat therapy, 197, 210

and movement, 196–197, 208–209
and oxygen, 99
therapies for, 209–212
expectations, 80

Farah, Mo, 97–98
fatigue, xxii, 13–14, 64, 120, 189
Felix, Antony, 223
fibromyalgia, xxii, 63–64
Finsen, Niels, 158
food, 181–185
in healthy diet, 37–39
nutrient absorption from, 28–29 (*see also* nourishment)
Food Rules (Pollan), 183
Fung, Jason, 183

Gebrselassie, Haile, 97
Gelfand, Amy, 125–126
genetic testing, 18–19
Goadsby, Peter, 125–126

Hamblin, Michael, 159–160, 164
happiness, 23–24, 69, 180
HbOT. *see* hyperbaric oxygen
headwinds, xviii, 24–36
disease and pain, 29–31
energy loss, 27–28
identifying your, 33–36
nutrient absorption, 28–29
time, 31–33
health. *see also specific areas of health, e.g.:* cognitive health
and dog ownership, 154
happiness and, 23–24
influences on, 36
with restricted eating, 184–185
as undemocratized, 32
heart health, 82–84, 88, 151
heat therapy, 79–95
and aging, 90–92
benefits of, 93–95
contrasting cold therapy and, 92–93

for exercise recovery, 197, 210
for heart health, 82–84
at home, 89
for mental and cognitive health, 84–87
and pain, 87–89
prior to stretching and exercise, 55–56
for sleep quality, 141–142
Henshaw, Nathaniel, 100
Herjavec, Robert, 60
high-intensity interval training (HIIT), 206
Hippocrates, xii, 77
holistic wellness, xvii, 6–9, 245
How To Stop Being Toxic (Felix), 223
Huberman, Andrew, 154
hydration, 119–133
and atrial fibrillation, 126–129
for chronic migraine, 122–126
for cognitive health, 129–130
dehydration, 121–122
and hydration budget, 132–133
hypohydration, xxii, 120
overhydration, 121, 131–132
hydration budget, 132–133
hyperbaric oxygen (HbOT), 99–105
for depression, 114
for long COVID, 106–108
for mental health, 110
mimicking effects of, 116–118
and mitochondrial function, 114–115
for sleep, 147–149
hyperhydration, 121, 131–132
hyper wellness, xvii, 1–24
addressing areas of concern in, 4–6
and age vs. aging, 9–13
challenges helped by, xxi–xxiii
evaluating therapies for, 230–238
improving your (*see* tailwinds)
journey toward, xix–xx, 228–230, 242–248
for living more, 23–24
obstacles to (*see* headwinds)
potential for, 13, 14
setting trajectory for, 13–14

hyper wellness (*cont.*)
    and "sick care" vs. holistic wellness, 6–9
    targets for, 20–22
    wellness census, 15–20
hypohydration, xxii, 120

immune function, 27, 40
    and cryotherapy, 68
    and heat therapy, 91
    and nourishment, 192, 193
    and oxygen, 99
improving your wellness. *see* tailwinds
IM (intramuscular) shots, 191–193
inflammation, xxii
    and cryotherapy, 62, 63, 68
    and heat therapy, 91, 93
    and IV drip therapy, 189
    and light therapy, 164, 211
initiating tailwinds, 36–37
injury recovery, xxii, 26
    with aging, 31, 204
    and movement, 204
    and oxygen, 99, 111
intramuscular (IM) shots, 191–193
"invisible gorilla" experiment, 16–17
involuntary muscle contraction, xxii, 57
IV drip therapy
    for atrial fibrillation, 128
    for cognitive health, 130
    for exercise recovery, 210–211
    for migraines, 120, 125–126
    for nutrient deficiencies, 187–191

James, LeBron, 211
Joel, Billy, 215
joint pain, xxii, 15–16, 21, 22
    and cryotherapy, 115–116, 240
    and hydration, 133
joint stiffness, xxii, 16, 21, 55–58
Joseph, Rich, 234

Kidd, Jason, 60
Kimball, Justin, 8

Knott, Maggie, 55, 56
Kuopio Ischaemic Heart Disease Risk
    Factor Study, 82, 83, 85

lack of time, xxii, 32, 34–36
Laukkanen, Jari, 82, 83, 85, 86, 94
Lewis, Gemma, 113–114
Li, Jun, 29
Lieberman, Matthew, 223
light, 153–176
    for brain health, 163–166
    for moods and mental health,
      161–163
    as most powerful tailwind, 175–176
    for muscle recovery and athletic
      performance, 171–172, 211
    from screens, 45–48
    for sexual health, 172–175
    for skin health, 167–171
    and sleep quality, 150–151
    unseen spectrum of, 156–160
long COVID, xxii, 106–108, 190
longevity, 12

McKeeman, Bruce, 104, 106
McKeeman, Judy, 104, 106
McNair, Jordan, 122
Mead, Sedgwick, 55, 56
medical exams, 17–18
meditation, 75
menopause, xxii, 240
mental fogginess, xxii, 64, 93, 99
mental health, 34–35
    assessing, 18
    and color, 157
    and cryotherapy, 69–71
    and dog ownership, 154
    and heat therapy, 6, 84–87, 94
    and light, 161–163
    and oxygen, 108–114
    and vegetable consumption, 38
migraine, xxiii, 122–126, 122–126
mitochondrial function, 27, 72, 114–115, 117

moods, xxiii, 16, 21
and color, 157
and heat therapy, 85
and hydration, 120
and light, 161–163, 168
and nourishment, 179–180
and sleep, 44
movement, 195–213. *see also* exercise
cryotherapy to maximize mobility,
55–58
and exercise recovery, 208–209
headwinds of, 199–201
motivation for, 201–205
need for, 212–213
tailwinds of, 198–199
vigorous exercise, 205–208
multiple sclerosis (MS), xxiii, 53–58
muscle pain, xxiii, 21–22
muscle recovery, 171–172, 211

NAD+, 34–35
Nightingale, Florence, 158
nourishment, 177–194
food, 181–185
IM shots for, 191–193
long-term impact of, 194
nutrient absorption, 28–29
supplementation, 185–194
nutrient absorption, 28–29, 34

obesity and weight, xxiii, 26, 40
benefits of small weight losses, 40
and cryotherapy, 240–241
and heat therapy, 80
and hydration, 126–127, 129
and movement, 195–197
and nourishment, 177–178,
181–185
during pandemic, 49
and sleep quality, 141, 142
The Obesity Code (Fung), 183
obstacles to wellness. *see* headwinds
overhydration, 121, 131–132

oxygen, 97–118
and cellular psychology, 114–118
hyperbaric, 99–104 (*see also*
hyperbaric oxygen [HbOT])
and long COVID, 106–108
and mental health, 108–114
"soft" hyperbaric chambers, 103–105

pain, 26
in cancer survivors, 30–31
chronic, xxi, 15–16, 26, 63–64, 79
and cryotherapy, 59
with excess weight, 40
and heat therapy, 87–89, 94
and hydration, 120, 133
as obstacle to wellness, 29–31
parasocial relationships, 217–218
Patrick, Rhonda, 91–92
peptides, 233–235
plantar fasciitis, xxiii, 80
Pollan, Michael, 183
postpartum fatigue, xxiii, 190
Priestley, Joseph, 100
Pritchett, Henry, 7–8
psoriasis, xxiii, 92, 167–169

rest, xvii. *see also* sleep
Restore Hyper Wellness, xiv–xvi, 11
Rideout, Ken, 9
Rymaszewska, Joanna, 69–70

safety of therapies, assessing, 230–238
saunas, 79–89, 92–94, 141–142. *see also*
heat therapy
screen time, 45–47, 137, 150, 200–201
secondary tailwinds, 37
Secret Book of the Physician, xii
sex drive, xxiii, 113, 172–175
Shakespeare, 13
Sheffield, Paul, 104
Sherr, Scott, 103
Shmerling, Robert, 189
"sick care" model, 6–9, 245

Sinclair, David, 93
skin, 54, 169–170
skin health, xxiii, 65–68, 79, 80, 167–171
sleep, xxiii, 46–47, 135–152
    and connection, 220
    and COVID-19 stress, 153
    and cryotherapy, 64, 65, 75, 240
    description and function of, 138–143
    and exercise, 41–42, 41–42
    and heat therapy, 85, 92
    and hydration, 127, 133
    and hyperbaric oxygen, 147–149,
       147–149
    and light sources, 45–48
    quality of, 135–138, 140–142
    tracking, 143–147, 143–147
    what sleep is, 138–143
    working at, 149–152, 149–152
sleep apnea, xxiii, 136, 136, 141–143
sleep hygiene, 45–47, 137–138, 150–152
The Sleep Solution (Winter), 136
Smith, Casey, 60
smoking, 11
"soft" hyperbaric chambers, 103–105
stress, xxiii
    during COVID-19 pandemic, 153
    and heat therapy, 79, 93
    and light therapy, 154–156, 166
    and nourishment, 190
stretching, 55–57, 196
Stringer Korey, 122
Sun, Nuo, 27
supplementation, 11, 28–29, 185–194

tailwinds, xviii, 24, 36–51
    eating habits, 37–41
    exercise, 41–44
    initiating and secondary, 36–37
    sleep, 44–48
    time management, 48–50
targets for hyper wellness, 20–22
TBI (traumatic brain injury), 163–164
Tei, Chuwa, 88

Thich Nhat Hanh, 117
time
    as headwind, xxii, 31–36
    as tailwind, 48–50
time-restricted eating, 184–185
traumatic brain injury (TBI), 163–164

ulcerative colitis, xxiii, 185–188
US Food and Drug Administration, 11,
    103–105, 234

Valtin, Heinz, 131, 132
virtuous cycle, xvii, 21, 22, 22, 228, 239–240

Walker, Matthew, 136, 150
watchpoints, 227–238
    assessing safety and success, 230–233
    evaluating interventions, 233–238
water, need for, 120–121. *see also*
  hydration
water intoxication, 132
waypoints of wellness, 238–242
wellness, xvii
    aging mitigated by, 12–13
    assessing your, 1–4, 15–20, 227–229
    gradual shifts in, 4–6
    holistic, xvii, 6–9, 245
    right-away (*see* hyper wellness)
wellness census, 15–20
whole-body cryotherapy, xi–xiv, 57,
    60–65, 67–70
Why We Sleep (Walker), 136
Więcek, Magdalena, 72–73
Willardson, Jeffrey, 202
willpower, 33
Winter, Chris, 136, 150
Wright, Ken, 175–176

Yamauchi, Toshiro, xii
Yaya Africa Athletics Village, 97, 98

Zhang, Jianfen, 129
Zhang, Na, 129

About the Authors

Jim Donnelly founded his first company in grad school, then spent time in the US military as an Army officer before marketing stints at brands including Kraft Foods, AT&T, Coca-Cola, and Citibank. In 2001, Jim leveraged his love for travel to build one of the most popular online travel communities in the world, IgoUgo.com, which earned a Webby Award for Best Travel Site in the US. After IgoUgo was sold to Sabre/Travelocity, Jim founded Pursuit Group, an incubator that launched high-end experiential retail businesses and one-of-a-kind boutique real estate projects.

Steve Welch started his first big entrepreneurial success, Mitos, in 2001 with hardly a cent to his name. Without ever raising outside money Steve built Mitos into a global company in the biotech manufacturing field prior to selling it in 2007 at the age of 30 to a Fortune 500 company. Under Steve's guidance, Mitos developed several critical innovations and patents that transformed the manufacturing process of biological drugs and vaccines and allowed Mitos to develop a global sales and distribution network.

Together Jim and Steve founded Restore Hyper Wellness, opening their first studio in 2015. From humble roots in the back office of that studio, new locations were added with therapies that include cryotherapy, IV nutrient supplementation, mild hyperbaric oxygen therapy, infrared saunas, compression, and red light therapy. In the process, the Restore team created an innovative new category of care, allowing clients to feel better and do more of what they love to do. Today, Restore Hyper Wellness has hundreds of locations across the country and is rapidly expanding.

Matthew D. LaPlante is an associate professor of journalism at Utah State University, where he teaches news reporting, narrative nonfiction writing, and crisis reporting. He has reported from more than a dozen nations, including Iraq, Cuba, Ethiopia, and El Salvador, and his work has appeared in the *Washington Post*, *Los Angeles Daily News*, CNN.com, and numerous other publications. LaPlante is the author of *Superlative: The Biology of Extremes* and cowriter of several books on the intersection of scientific discovery and society.